End of Life Care

D1335527

End of Life Care

362.175

48

End of Life Care

A Care Worker Handbook

Caroline Morris and Fiona Collier

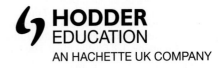

HODDER
EDUCATION
AN HACHETTE UK COMPANY

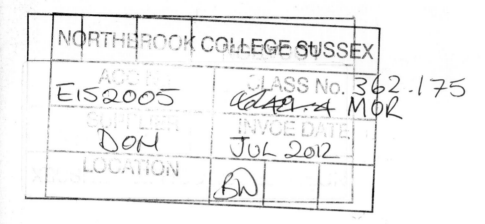

NORTHBROOK COLLEGE SUSSEX

ACC E152005 CLASS No. 362.175 MOR

SUPPLIER DON INVOICE DATE JUL 2012

LOCATION BW

Orders: please contact Bookpoint Ltd, 130 Milton Park, Abingdon, Oxon
OX14 4SB. Telephone: (44) 01235 827720. Fax: (44) 01235 400454. Lines are
open from 9.00–5.00, Monday to Saturday, with a 24 hour message
answering service. You can also order through our website
www.hoddereducation.co.uk

If you have any comments to make about this, or any of our other titles,
please send them to educationenquiries@hodder.co.uk

British Library Cataloguing in Publication Data
A catalogue record for this title is available from the British Library

ISBN: 978 1 444 16324 7

First Edition Published 2012
Impression number   10 9 8 7 6 5 4 3 2 1
Year   2016 2015 2014 2013 2012

Copyright © 2012 Caroline Morris and Fiona Collier

All rights reserved. No part of this publication may be reproduced or
transmitted in any form or by any means, electronic or mechanical,
including photocopy, recording, or any information storage and retrieval
system, without permission in writing from the publisher or under licence
from the Copyright Licensing Agency Limited. Further details of such
licences (for reprographic reproduction) may be obtained from the
Copyright Licensing Agency Limited, of Saffron House, 6–10 Kirby Street,
London EC1N 8TS.

Hachette UK's policy is to use papers that are natural, renewable and
recyclable products and made from wood grown in sustainable forests.
The logging and manufacturing processes are expected to conform to the
environmental regulations of the country of origin.

Artwork by Barking Dog Art
Cover photo © deanm 1974/Fotolia.com
Typeset by Pantek Media, Maidstone, Kent.
Printed and bound in Italy for Hodder Education, an Hachette UK
Company, 338 Euston Road, London NW1 3BH

Contents

Acknowledgements and author biographies

Acknowledgements

Every effort has been made to trace and acknowledge ownership of copyright. The publishers will be glad to make suitable arrangements with any copyright holders whom it has not been possible to contact.

Photo credits

Figure 2.1 © gilles lougassi – Fotolia.com; Figure 2.3 © Elenathewise – Fotolia.com; Figure 2.4 © Tetra Images/Alamy; Figure 2.6 © Corbis Super RF/Alamy; Figure 3.1 © Yuri Arcurs – Fotolia.com; Figure 4.1 © Radius Images/Alamy; Figure 4.2 (left) © Tadeusz Ibrom – Fotolia.com; Figure 4.2 (right) © fisfra – Fotolia.com; Figure 4.4 © Shawn Hempel – Fotolia.com; Figure 5.5 © Blend Images/Alamy; Figure 6.4 © Alexander Raths – Fotolia.com; Figure 6.8 © John Birdsall/Photofusion; Figure 7.1 © Roman Milert – Fotolia.com; Figure 7.2 © A ROOM WITH VIEWS/Alamy; Figure 7.5 © Sharon McTeir; Figure 7.6 © gilles lougassi – Fotolia.com; Figure 8.2 © David J. Green/Alamy; Figure 8.4 © gunnar3000 – Fotolia.com; Figure 8.5 © nyul – Fotolia.com.

Author biographies

Caroline Morris has a background in the health services, having worked as a nurse, Registered Care Manager and, more recently, a teacher, lecturer and Education Consultant, delivering in Health and Social Care since 1992. Caroline has provided services to OCR, Edexcel, OfQual, OU and EDI as an external verifier/Consultant in Public Services since 1997, and has been involved in writing materials and specifications for publishers and EDI and OCR awarding bodies. Caroline is carrying out post-graduate research in education to achieve PhD, and also undertakes inspections on behalf of EDI, OU and BAC.

Fiona Collier is a registered nurse with a varied experience of providing end of life care within the intensive care environment. In addition to her clinical experience Fiona has also developed her skills as a teacher, trainer and internal moderator within Further Education providing work based training and education to staff working in health and social care environments. Fiona is presently working as a Consultant in Education and Training for the Health and Social Care Sector where she develops, delivers and evaluates training as well as writing educational material for publishers and awarding bodies.

Walkthrough

We want you to succeed!

This book has been designed to include all the topic knowledge, assessment support and practical advice you will need for the following qualifications:

- Level 2 Award in End of Life Care
- Level 2 Certificate in End of Life Care
- Level 3 Award in End of Life Care
- Level 3 Certificate in End of Life Care

The book has been written with the work-based learner in mind. Everything in it reflects the assessment criteria and evidence based approach that is applied to this vocational qualification.

In the pages that follow you will find up-to-date resource material which will develop your knowledge, rehearse your skills and help you to gain your qualification.

Prepare for what you are going to cover in this unit, and prepare for assessment:

The reading and activities in this chapter will help you to:

- Understand the principles of advance care planning
- Understand the person centred approach to advance care planning
- Understand when advance care planning may be required

Reinforce concepts with hands-on learning and generate evidence for assignments

Time to reflect

2.1 Experience of personal grief, your feelings and the support you accessed

If you have experienced personal grief what feelings did you have? What support, if any, did you access?

Reinforce concepts with hands-on learning and generate evidence for assignments

Evidence activity

 4.5 Practitioners accessed in your service

Review the practitioners accessed in your service. Are there unmet needs? If so, which practitioners could support these?

■ Research and investigate

 3.1 Find out about the key outcomes of Lord Darzi's review

What were the key outcomes of Lord Darzi's review?

Understand how your learning fits into real life and your working environment

Case Study

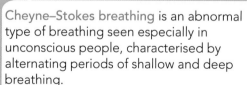

5.5 Shamus

Shamus is an 87-year-old gentleman who lives in a residential care setting. He has lived in the home for seven years and is receiving end of life care, as his health has been deteriorating. When Shamus dies, the senior staff at the home make a decision not to tell the other service users.

Explain the possible consequences of these actions.

Check new words and what they mean

Key terms

Cheyne–Stokes breathing is an abnormal type of breathing seen especially in unconscious people, characterised by alternating periods of shallow and deep breathing.

You've just covered a whole unit so here's a guide to what assessors will be looking for and links to activities that can help impress them

Assessment summary

Your reading of this chapter and completion of the activities will have prepared you to demonstrate your learning and understanding of end of life care. To achieve this unit, your assessor will require you to:

Learning outcomes	Assessment criteria
Learning outcome **1**: Understand the effects of symptoms in relation to end of life care:	**1.1** Identify a range of conditions where you might provide end of life care See Evidence activity 1.1, p.30
	1.2 Identify common symptoms associated with end of life care See Evidence activity 1.2, p.31
Learning outcome **2**: Be able to manage symptoms of end of life care:	**2.1** Demonstrate a range of techniques to provide symptom relief See Evidence activity 2.1, p.37
	2.2 Describe own role in supporting therapeutic options used in symptom relief See Evidence activity 2.2, p.40

For Unit EOL 301

Understand how to provide support when working in end of life care

What are you finding out?

Many people believe that end of life care is only applicable to supporting people in the final hours of their life. This is certainly not the case. End of life care is aimed at helping those with advanced, progressive illness to live as well as possible until they die. It focuses on preparing for the anticipated death and managing care to ensure comfort, in addition to providing a high standard of care during and around the time of death, and immediately afterwards.

End of life care is no longer confined to specialist services, but includes the support and care given by health and social care workers in all care settings. It is therefore important that every person who works in an environment which provides end of life care is aware of the emotive issues surrounding death and dying.

The reading and activities in this chapter will help you to:

- Understand current approaches to end of life care

- Understand an individual's response to their anticipated death

- Understand factors regarding communication for those involved in end of life care

- Understand how to support those involved in end of life care situations

- Understand how the symptoms might be identified in end of life care

- Understand advance care planning.

LO1 Understand current approaches to end of life care

1.1 Analyse the impact of national and local drivers on current approaches to end of life care

In the past, the profile of end of life care has been relatively low within the NHS and social care services. Reflecting this, outside of hospice settings the standard of care has been inconsistent and variable. Standards have been good in some areas of care but not in others. This has led to a situation where some people have had a good experience at the end of their life whilst others have not. In addition, end of life care has been seen as a specialist area of care being provided primarily to individuals who have received a diagnosis of cancer.

In response to these inconsistencies, the Department of Health launched its first ever strategy for end of life care in 2008. The end of life care strategy is a ten year initiative aiming to improve the quality of care for all adults facing the end of their life, regardless of age, gender, ethnicity, religious beliefs, disability, sexual orientation, diagnosis or social status; and to provide them with more choice about where they would like to live, die and be cared for.

In order to achieve its aims, the end of life care strategy outlines ten key objectives. These are to:

1. Increase public awareness and discussion of death and dying. This will make it easier for people to discuss their own preferences around end of life care and should also act as a driver to improve overall service quality

2. Ensure that all people are treated with dignity and respect at the end of their lives

3. Ensure that pain and suffering amongst people approaching the end of life are kept to an absolute minimum with access to skilful symptom management for optimum quality of life

4. Ensure that all those approaching the end of life have access to physical, psychological, social and spiritual care

5. Ensure that people's individual needs, priorities and preferences for end of life care are identified, documented, reviewed, respected and acted upon wherever possible

6. Ensure that the many services people need are well coordinated, so that patients receive seamless care

7. Ensure that high quality care is provided in the last days of life and after death in all care settings

8. Ensure that carers are appropriately supported both during a patient's life and in bereavement

9. Ensure that health and social care professionals at all levels are provided with the necessary education and training to enable them to provide high quality care

10. Ensure that services provide good value for money for the taxpayer.

Source: http://www.cpa.org.uk/cpa/ End_of_Life_Care_Strategy.pdf

Integral to the success of the end of life care strategy is the development of a care pathway for end of life care. A care pathway provides a means of mapping the route that a person will take from their first contact with health services to the completion of their treatment or care.

Although it recognises that each person's experience of death and dying is unique, the end of life care pathway consists of six steps and was developed to help individuals providing health and social care to people nearing the end of life (see Figure 1.1). The Care Pathway aims to ensure that high quality, person-centred care is provided which is well planned, coordinated and monitored while being responsive to the individual's needs and wishes. It is important to be aware of this pathway as health and social care settings providing end of life care must demonstrate that they are supporting its implementation.

Running alongside the six steps, the end of life care strategy emphasises the importance of ensuring health and social care services also provide:

- support for families and carers
- information for service users and carers
- spiritual care for service users and families
- social care for service users and families.

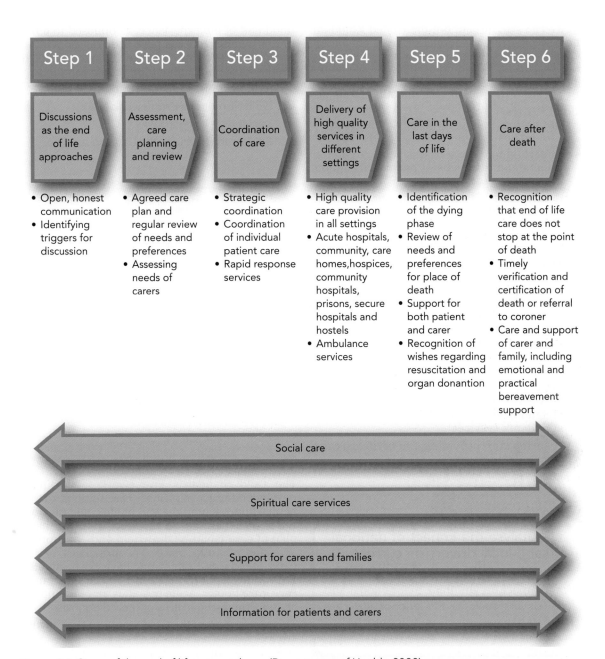

Figure 1.1 Steps of the end of life care pathway (Department of Health, 2008)

The National End of Life Care Programme document 'The route to success in end of life care – achieving quality in care homes' (2010) was developed to provide information about what should be included in the process of good end of life care delivery. The route to success follows the six steps of the pathway laid out in the National Strategy and includes questions for staff and managers to ask themselves about the end of life care provision in their care home.

In January 2009 the Department of Health published the NHS Constitution. This set out the rights and responsibilities of the people of England with regard to the NHS. The Constitution itself says:

"The NHS … is there to improve our health and well-being, supporting us to keep mentally and physically well, to get better when we are ill and, when we cannot fully recover, to stay as well as we can to the end of our lives."

So we can see, throughout the United Kingdom, there is presently a national drive to encourage all care settings to implement ways of ensuring best practice in providing care for people with a life limiting illness. At local levels, health and social care organisations are initiating strategies aimed at:

- promoting public awareness about issues around death, dying and end of life care
- undertaking needs assessments to better understand the needs of people throughout the end of life care pathway
- develop commissioning plans for end of life care covering all chronic conditions
- using the nationally recognised tools, such as the Liverpool Care Pathway, Preferred Priorities of Care or the Gold Standards Framework approach, to ensure the needs and preferences of those approaching end of life are assessed
- ensuring information is available on individuals who are approaching the end of life including the care plan, preferred place of care and any advance directives where appropriate
- ensuring appropriate information is shared between relevant services, for example out of hours, the Emergency Department and ambulance services
- ensuring staff providing end of life care are competent to do so.

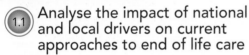

Evidence activity

1.1 **Analyse the impact of national and local drivers on current approaches to end of life care**

What impact do you think that national and local drivers such as the end of life care strategy has had on current approaches to end of life care?

1.2 **Evaluate how a range of tools for end of life care can support the individual and others**

In order to help providers of care meet the objectives of the end of life care strategy and to ensure people accessing end of life care experience a good end of life experience, as opposed to a bad one, a number of tools have been developed and are currently being used by numerous health professionals throughout the United Kingdom.

Three of the most well-known tools are the:

- Gold Standards Framework (GSF)
- Liverpool Care Pathway (LCP)
- Preferred Priorities for Care document.

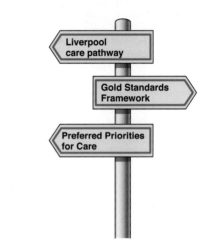

Figure 1.2 End of life care tools

The Gold Standards Framework

The Gold Standards Framework was initially developed for use in primary care settings so that people approaching the end of life could be identified, their care needs assessed, in order that a plan of care could be drawn up and appropriate agencies put into place. The principles of the Gold Standards Framework have been adapted for various settings and can be used in primary care, care homes, acute hospitals, prisons and for all individuals regardless of their diagnosis.

The overall aims of the Gold Standard Framework are to:

- improve the quality of care for individuals who are nearing the end of their lives
- improve coordination and collaboration with all members of the care team
- reduce the number of people who are unnecessarily transferred to hospital in the last stages of life.

The Gold Standards Framework involves three steps that are facilitated by effective and clear communication. It aims to:

1. Identify people in need of end of life care.
2. Assess and record the needs and preferences of the individual.
3. Plan and provide care appropriate to the individual's needs.

The five goals of the Gold Standard Framework aim to ensure:

1. The service user's symptoms are controlled.
2. The service user is enabled to choose their preferred priorities for care and where they would like to spend the last phase of their life.
3. The service user feels safe and secure, with fewer episodes of crisis.
4. The carers feel supported, involved, empowered and satisfied.
5. There is enhanced confidence and teamwork among the carers and communication and collaboration with other professionals are maximised.

In order to achieve these objectives, the Gold Standard Framework has established seven core standards; also known as the seven Cs. These are shown in Table 1.1.

The Liverpool Care Pathway

The Liverpool Care Pathway was established by a specialist palliative care team at the Royal Liverpool and Broadgreen University Hospitals and the team at the Liverpool Marie Curie Centre. The aim of the team was to develop a pathway that health professionals could follow in the last days or hours of a person's life. The Liverpool Care Pathway is therefore a tool that can be used for all people who are in their last days of life, irrespective of their primary disease or the cause of their imminent death.

The Liverpool Care Pathway for the Dying person was developed to transfer the hospice model of care into other care settings. It is recognised nationally and internationally as leading practice in care of the dying to enable people to die a dignified death and provide support to their relatives and carers.

The Liverpool Care Pathway provides guidance on the different aspects of care, including:

- comfort measures
- symptom control

- anticipatory prescribing of medication and the discontinuation of inappropriate interventions
- emotional and spiritual support
- communication with the dying person and their loved ones
- communication with the Primary Health Care Team.

Preferred Priorities for Care

The 'Preferred Priorities for Care' is a person-held document and was designed to facilitate choice in relation to end of life care. It can help individuals who are living with a life-limiting illness to prepare for their future. It gives them an opportunity to think about, talk about and write down their preferences and priorities for care at the end of their life.

The Preferred Priorities for Care can help carers to understand what is important to the individual when planning care. If a time comes when, for whatever reason, the individual is unable to make a decision for themselves, anyone who has to make decisions about care on the individual's behalf will have to take into account anything the person has written in their Preferred Priorities for Care. The document is updated as required and travels with the individual throughout their pathway of care.

Evidence activity

 Evaluate how a range of tools for end of life care can support the individual and others

While maintaining confidentiality, undertake a case study relating to an individual who is approaching the end of their life within your workplace. Evaluate how one of the end of life tools you are using has/can be used to support this person and their family.

How does this tool support the care being delivered by the staff? What are its strengths and what are its weaknesses?

NORTHBROOK COLLEGE SUSSEX
LEARNING RESOURCE CENTRE
LIBRARY

Table 1.1 Core standards of the Gold Standard Framework

The seven core standards of the Gold Standard Framework are:	
C1: Communication	Care settings using the Gold Standards Framework maintain a Supportive Care Register to record, plan and evaluate the care of people who are receiving end of life care. The register is also used to facilitate discussions surrounding the person's care within regular team meetings.
C2: Coordination	Each team should have a nominated person to coordinate and oversee the organisation and smooth running of the framework.
C3: Control of symptoms	Every person requiring end of life care should have their symptoms and any associated problems assessed, recorded, discussed and acted upon in accordance with the agreed strategy. The control of symptoms should take into account emotional, social, psychological and spiritual needs as well as physical.
C4: Continuity of care	Continuity of care includes out-of-hours care and staff should be aware of what help is available out of hours and how speedily this can be accessed. This is important in helping to prevent unnecessary admissions to hospital. The person and immediate family should be provided with a pack, which details important telephone numbers and a 'who's who', in addition to what to do and who to contact in an emergency.
C5: Continued learning	In order to provide a high standard of end of life care, staff must be given the opportunity to access resources to keep their knowledge and skills up to date. Staff must also be given the opportunity to discuss, learn from and reflect on their experiences, in order to identify areas of best practice and also to identify areas for further development.
C6: Carer support	Supporting carers is an essential part of end of life care. Practical and emotional support should be made available to carers throughout the process of caring and also in the form of bereavement care following the death of their loved one.
C7: Care in the dying phase	C7 is a natural extension of the other six core standards. Every person entering the final days of life must be appropriately cared for. This is the time when non-essential drug interventions are discontinued. Care focuses on ensuring the person is as comfortable as possible and ensuring spiritual and emotional needs are being met. The Gold Standards Framework recommends the implementation of the Liverpool Care Pathway at this point.

1.3 Analyse the stages of the local end of life care pathway

At a very basic level a care pathway is a plan of how someone should be cared for when they have a particular medical condition or set of symptoms. Doctors, nurses and other health professionals record the care that they give in the care pathway document. This ensures that their notes are all kept together, in the same place, and everyone involved knows what is going on. The care pathway should always:

- involve the service user and their carers
- focus on the service user and their family
- clearly set out the standards for how things should be done
- involve all professionals caring for the patient and their family.

The care pathway should be agreed by all the people involved in caring for the service user. It should detail the service user's journey and should help ensure individuals receive appropriate care in accordance with their individual needs. The care pathway aims to predict possible problems that the person may experience, and hopefully prevent them before they occur.

The End of Life Care Pathway was developed as a result of the End of Life Care Strategy set out by the Government in 2008. The End of Life Care Pathway aims to ensure that high-quality, person-centred care is provided that is well planned, coordinated and monitored, while being responsive to the individual's needs and wishes and consists of the following steps:

- identification of people approaching the end of life and initiating discussions about preferences for end of life care
- assessing and agreeing a care plan, which details the individual's needs and preferences and reviewing these on a regular basis
- coordination of care
- delivery of high-quality services
- management of the last days of life
- care after death
- support for carers, both during a person's illness and after that person's death.

Case Study

(1.3) **Application of the End of Life Care Pathway**

Mr Collinson, a 69-year-old gentleman, has been diagnosed with Motor Neurone Disease following a period of general weakness, slurred speech and a heavy feeling in his arms. He lives with his wife and has taken the diagnosis very well. Some would say he is almost in denial. Mr and Mrs Collinson have no other family around; however, they do have very helpful neighbours. They live in a bungalow and up until now Mr Collinson has been very fit and independent. Not long after his diagnosis, Mr Collinson developed difficulty swallowing but didn't want to have a feeding tube inserted. He wanted to stay at home and refused to be admitted to hospital.

How could the End of Life Care Pathway be applied to Mr Collinson at this stage of his illness.

Evidence activity

(1.3) **Analyse the stages in the End of Life Care Pathway**

You are required to give a talk on the End of Life Care Pathway. Make a poster which clearly explains the stages in the End of Life Care Pathway.

LO2 Understand an individual's response to their anticipated death

2.1 Evaluate models of loss and grief

There are many models which explain grief and loss. Models are helpful when supporting people through bereavement because they provide a framework for us to see how people who are bereaved are experiencing grief and then to consider how we can help them. The following are some common models of grief.

Colin Murray Parkes Model: Phases of grief

The Colin Murray Parkes model of grief advocates that many people who are bereaved will experience grief in phases and will work through these stages at their own pace.

Initially the individual will experience shock which may show itself in many different ways, for example numbness or disbelief. Following this stage, the individual will experience separation and pain which may show itself in waves of distress, intense yearning for the person who has died and feelings of emptiness. The next stage is that of despair, which may manifest itself in depression, difficulties with concentration, anger, guilt and restlessness. Once the individual has worked through these stages he or she will finally reach the stage of acceptance.

William Worden Model: Tasks of mourning

Worden suggested that people need to work through their reactions in order to make a complete adjustment. Within Worden's tasks of bereavement, grief is considered to consist of four overlapping areas and the individual must work through each of these emotions. In order to accept the reality of the loss the individual must:

- accept the reality of the loss
- work through the pain of grief
- adjust to an environment in which the person who has died is missing
- emotionally relocate the person who has died and move on with life.

Stroebe and Schut Model: Dual process model

Stroebe and Schut advocate that you cannot neatly package grief work into stages which need to be worked through. Their model describes feelings and activities following bereavement which encompass loss and restoration. They see that both kinds of activities are very important in order for an individual to 'recover' from bereavement. When a person is bereaved they may move back and forth between the loss and restoration from the beginning of their loss. Loss activities include grief work, intrusion of grief and denial or avoidance of restoration activities. Restoration orientated activities include attending to the changes arising from the death, doing new things and taking on new roles and identity.

Elisabeth Kübler Ross: Five stages model

According to Kübler Ross, there are five stages that a dying person goes through when faced with a life limiting diagnosis. The five stages progress from denial through to acceptance. Whilst the work of Kübler Ross related to the experiences of people who are dying, it has been adapted by other authors and used as a means of describing grief work in a more generally. The stages are outlined in Table 1.2.

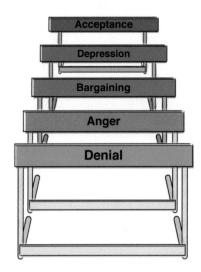

Figure 1.3 Stages of grief

Table 1.2 Stages of grief of a dying person

5 stages of grief of a dying person	
Stage 1: Denial and isolation	Denial can manifest itself through emotions of shock and disbelief. There may be feelings associated with numbness. The person may feel as though this is a dream and that what they are experiencing is not true.
Stage 2: Anger	Following the denial stage, the individual will come to terms with the reality of what is happening to them and the feelings associated with denial may lead to intense feelings of anger. Anger can manifest itself in several ways. The person may feel resentful and rage at what they are faced with. They may question 'why me?'
Stage 3: Bargaining	This is a stage where individuals begin to adjust to their goals, hopes and expectations. The person may attempt to negotiate the situation either with another person or with God. This stage often involves promises of better behaviour or significant life change which will be made in exchange for the reversal of the loss.

5 stages of grief of a dying person	
Stage 4: Depression	Once the realisation that the situation is not reversible sinks in, the individual often sinks into a depression. It is within this stage that the individual realises the inevitability of what is happening to them. The reality of the impending loss and the irreversibility sinks in. It is within this stage that grieving people begin to cry and experience difficulties with sleeping or eating.
Stage 5: Acceptance	This is the stage where the individual comes to terms with what is happening. Kübler Ross acknowledges that if a person has enough time, and has been given support in working through the stages of grief, they will reach a stage where they can finally come to terms with what is happening to them.

These stages are not rigid. They are guidelines and Elisabeth Kübler Ross gives emphasis to the fact that they can occur in any order and at any time. They can also happen simultaneously.

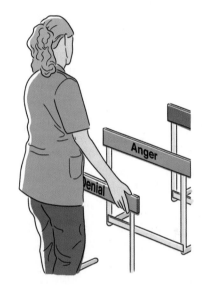

Figure 1.4 Grief support

Evidence activity

2.1 Evaluate models of loss and grief

Evaluate two models of grief and state the differences between the models.

2.2 Describe how to support the individual throughout each stage of grief

The first step in supporting a person through the stages of grief is to realise that every person is different, with their own set of values and mechanisms for coping. Supporting a person who is nearing the end of their life can be very difficult. It may be difficult to know what to say to the person, or to know how to react to the various emotions the person may express.

Steps that can be taken to support the individual are given in Table 1.3.

Evidence activity

2.2 Supporting a person at each stage of grief

Describe how you might support a person at each stage of grief.

Table 1.3 Providing support for individuals throughout each stage of grief

Stage of grief	Steps that can be taken to support the individual
Stage 1: Denial and isolation	<ul><li>Give the person time to go over the same ground again and again</li><li>Accept the feelings of denial, try not to contradict the person by trying to make them come to terms with reality</li><li>Remain non-judgemental no matter how critical the person may be of the care they are receiving</li><li>Be prepared for extreme swings in mood; these are natural at this stage</li><li>Respect that the person may need space and may not wish to talk at this stage</li><li>If you or the person are finding talking openly difficult encourage the person to speak with someone else, for example, their GP or a nurse</li></ul>
Stage 2: Anger	<ul><li>Do not take anger personally; although it may appear to be, it is not directly aimed at you</li><li>Acknowledge the validity of the person's feelings. Never ignore or dismiss the person's anger</li><li>Encourage the person to discuss their feelings. This is important in order to enable the person to move on to the next stage</li><li>Empathise with the person. Try to put yourself in the person's shoes</li><li>Ensure you promote choice and independence, as the anger may come from a loss of control</li><li>Be understanding and patient</li><li>Encourage the person to reflect on their feelings and what helped them to cope with feelings of anger in the past</li><li>Let the person know that what they are feeling is acceptable and 'normal'</li></ul>
Stage 3: Bargaining	<ul><li>Encourage the person to talk about their feelings, their hopes and aspirations. Although a person may not be able to hope for recovery, they may still hope for other things and, as long as those hopes are realistic, bargaining can help them to maintain a degree of hope</li><li>Discuss with the person how they may be able to achieve their hopes and what support may be needed to fulfil their aspirations</li><li>Ensure the rest of the care team are made aware of the person's wishes and ensure that any documentation is kept up to date to ensure the person's hopes and aspirations are recorded</li></ul>
Stage 4: Depression	<ul><li>Take time to listen to the person; this is a very important aspect of supporting a person who is suffering from depression</li><li>Create an atmosphere that will encourage the person to open up to you; for example, offer the person a cup of tea</li><li>Empathise with the person's feelings. Acknowledge the pain the person is feeling, but do not rush in with words of advice</li><li>Where appropriate, offer hope. This is very important, as this will help to improve the person's sense of well-being</li><li>Respect the person's choices, as not all people will want to talk</li><li>Report and document any conversations you have with the individual to facilitate continuity of care</li></ul>
Stage 5: Acceptance	<ul><li>Help loved ones to come to terms with the acceptance as they may feel rejected, especially if the individual becomes detached from what is going on</li><li>Support the person to fulfil any final wishes</li></ul>

2.3 **Explain the need to explore with each individual their own specific areas of concern as they face death**

It is easy to back away from discussing a service user's fears and concerns as they face the end of life. This is often due to concerns about opening up a can of worms, or being unable to deal with what we may discuss. It is, however, an essential aspect of care and is necessary in supporting a person to die with a peaceful and untroubled mind. This aspect of care is just as important as supporting a person with their physical needs.

Evidence activity

2.3 Explain the need to explore with each individual their own specific areas of concern as they face death

Why do you think it is important to explore specific areas of concern with individuals as they face the end of their life?

2.4 **Describe how an individual's awareness of spirituality may change as they approach end of life**

Spirituality is whatever gives a person meaning, value and worth in their life. This may not necessarily be an organised religion or god. It is the strength and solace people gain from things that are important to them that give a person a purpose to living. It may be the love of their family, the peace of the countryside or enjoying creating a piece of art. Spirituality ultimately relates to the individual ways a person finds connection and meaning in life.

As people approach the end of their life, they may encounter spiritual questions and conflicts, issues of meaning and significance, questions of an appropriate death, and challenges to their spiritual assumptions and/or beliefs or hopes about what occurs during and after death.

Evidence activity

 2.4 Describe how an individual's awareness of spirituality may change as they approach end of life

Think about your own spirituality and the things that are spiritually important to you. How do you think your awareness of these spiritually important things may change if you were approaching the end of your life?

LO3 Understand factors regarding communication for those involved in end of life care

3.1 **Explain the principles of effective listening and information giving, including the importance of picking up on cues and non-verbal communication**

Effective communication is a two-way process. It involves an exchange of thoughts, views, feelings or emotions, through speaking, listening and observing.

Within the field of end of life care, communication is:

- a process used for exchanging information between service users, their family, carers, and health and social care professionals
- underpinned by mutual understanding, respect and awareness of peoples' roles and functions
- the process through which service users, their family and carers are helped to explore issues and arrive at decisions.

We constantly communicate with each other and as we communicate we use all of our senses.

Developing effective listening skills is just as important as developing your speaking skills. Effective communication is a two-way process, and without effective listening skills, meaningful communication will be lessened.

Listening to people involves more than just hearing what they say. To listen well you need to be able to hear the words being spoken, think about what the words mean, then think about how you are going to respond to the person. You can also demonstrate that you are listening through your body language and facial expressions. For example, if you are yawning and looking round the room when a person is talking, you may give the impression that you are bored and uninterested. By shaking your head and frowning, you may give the impression that you disapprove of what is being said.

Good communication is not just about what is said, but also about what we hear. All too often we can be too busy talking when we should be listening. One of the best ways to communicate with people who are nearing the end of their life is to stop talking and start listening. Listening, however, is more than not talking. Listening involves not only hearing what is being said but also attempting to understand what lies behind the words spoken.

Effective listening requires a continuous determined effort to pay attention to the person who is speaking and to the words that are being spoken. Listening is not easy and is not the same as hearing.

Listening is not a natural process. Listening involves paying attention, remembering and understanding the content of what the person who is speaking has said. Hearing, however, is a natural process as one does not have to learn to hear. Listening is by far the most important of all communication skills. It does not come naturally to most people, so we need to work hard at it to stop ourselves 'jumping in' and giving our opinions.

'Active listening' is a 'person-centred' communication skill, based on the work of psychologist Carl Rogers, which involves giving free and undivided attention to the service user.

Active listening

Active listening involves much more than simply hearing what another person is saying. To listen actively you must:

- give the person your full attention
- try to understand exactly what the person is trying to communicate
- help the person to express themselves.

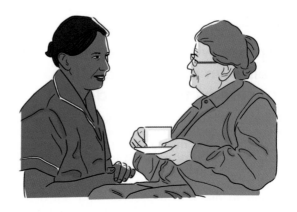

Figure 1.5 Active listening

 # Research and investigate

 Observe your colleagues whilst they are communicating with other people within your workplace. Make a note of any active listening skills your colleagues use when they are communicating.

The skills of active listening involve:

- **Time** – it is essential that time is made in order to ensure you can focus the whole of your attention on the individual and what they are communicating to you. This will allow you to focus on and respond to the person's feelings, needs, hopes and fears.

- **Giving the person your full attention** – this means focusing on the person, with openness and respect, whilst putting your own concerns and thoughts to one side. Observing the person's non-verbal communication as well as listening to everything the person is saying will help you to interpret the messages lying behind the person's words and behaviour.

- **Offering minimal prompts** – for example, nodding your head or making affirming sounds such as 'yes' or 'I see' will indicate to the person that you are listening and that you are interested.

- **Repeating and paraphrasing** – either using the person's own words, or finding your own words to represent what you think the person means, for example "so you are saying you are worried" will indicate to the person that you are actively listening.

- **Reflecting feelings** – noticing feelings that the person indicates verbally or non-verbally and mentioning these, for example, "you sound angry" or "you look very sad".

- **Mirroring** – observing the other person's body language and picking up on the person's non-verbal cues can assist in ensuring your own body language reflects the other person's body language. If, for example, the person is hunched over, upset or crying, you might lean forward and show a sad facial expression.

- **Focusing** – if necessary, focusing is about finding an appropriate moment to take a conversation back and focus in on an area of significance such as something mentioned, or a feeling demonstrated by the other person, for example, "when you spoke about your grandchildren, you looked very sad…".

- **Questioning** – when you are actively listening, you might ask questions mainly to help the person expand on what they are saying. For example, "You said you didn't want your family to know how upset you are … can you tell me why?" or "You said you didn't want to be a burden … can you tell me why you think you are a burden?". You might also need to ask questions to clarify that you've understood the person correctly.

- **Look for the feelings behind the words** – A good active listener will not only hear the words a person is saying, but will search for the feelings or meanings behind the words. Equally, a person may express hidden fears within buried questions. This is where a person asks a question or makes a comment whilst you are talking. It is important that these questions and statements are not ignored as they can be very significant.

- **Summarising** – when appropriate, re-capping on a section of a conversation or at the end of the conversation to ensure you have understood the person's key messages.

- **Silence** – being quiet at the appropriate moment can give the person the time they need to gather their thoughts and express what is important for them.

A good active listener will not only hear the content of what is being said but will also hear the intent or feelings contained within the words and tone of voice.

Non-verbal communication

To be an effective communicator, you have to notice how other people respond to your communication. People react non-verbally both to the way that you are communicating with them and to the content of your communication. You can therefore obtain feedback through the person's body language. Indeed, this may be the only kind of response you receive from some people who are not confident enough or who are too unwell to speak to you.

Non-verbal communication refers to the messages we send out to express ideas and opinions without talking. It has been said that as much as 80% of our communication is expressed through non-verbal means. Non-verbal communication, otherwise known as body language, is a vital form of communication. When we interact with other people, we continuously give and receive wordless signals. All of our non-verbal behaviours, including the gestures we make, the way we sit, how close we stand, how much eye contact we make, all send strong messages to the other person. For example, the way you listen, look, move, and react tell the other person whether or not you care and how well you're listening. The non-verbal signals you send either produce a sense of interest, trust, and desire for connection. On the other hand, they can generate disinterest, distrust and confusion.

Non-verbal communication can be extremely important for individuals who are living with a life limiting illness, especially if the ability to communicate verbally is limited. These people will rely on methods of non-verbal communication in order to make their needs and feelings known to other people.

We already know that communication is a two way process. It is important that members of staff have a good knowledge of the power of non-verbal communication and use their observational skills in order to interpret what the other person is trying to communicate through their body language.

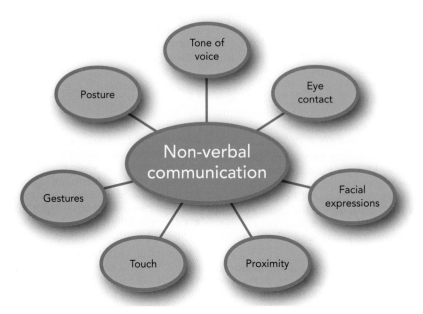

Figure 1.6 The main elements of non-verbal communication

Tone of voice

The tone of your voice can say a lot more than the words you choose. Your tone of voice is capable of communicating many different things, for example, if you are feeling upset, irritated, bored or angry. Care and attention must be taken as other people may pick up on your feelings through the tone of your voice.

There may be times, however, when you intend to communicate through the tone of your voice. For example, you may wish to let other members of the team know that you are annoyed about a certain situation in order that an issue can be addressed.

Eye contact

Eye contact is an essential element of non-verbal communication. Eye contact can establish where your focus is. If an individual is talking to you and you are looking all over the room, it is very unlikely that you are giving the conversation 100% of your attention. Equally, maintaining eye contact can convey interest and encourage the other person to show interest in your conversation. It is, however, important to ensure eye contact remains natural. It is important to blink naturally as staring can be interpreted as being aggressive.

We can sometimes interpret thoughts and feelings through eye to eye contact. The eyes are particularly expressive in communicating joy, sadness, anger, fear or confusion. We can often tell what someone is feeling by their eyes. Our eyes become wider when we are excited or happy.

It is important to keep your eyes at the same level as the other person's eyes in order not to appear authoritative. This can be achieved by sitting down with the person.

Facial expressions

The human face is incredibly expressive. We are able to express countless emotions without saying a single word, and unlike some forms of non-verbal communication, facial expressions are universal. The facial expressions for happiness, sadness, anger, surprise, fear and disgust are the same across differing cultures.

Facial expressions are often used to convey meaning when communicating. In fact, the face is perhaps the most important channel of emotional information. A face can light up with enthusiasm, energy and approval, express confusion or boredom, and can also scowl with displeasure. A smile can show happiness and a frown can communicate annoyance.

Having the ability to read facial expressions is a very important tool when communicating with people who are nearing the end of their life. Very often it is easy to observe how a person is feeling through their facial expressions.

Proximity and personal space

Proximity refers to the distance that is maintained between people throughout the process of communication. It is concerned with 'personal space'. This is a really important aspect of communication as this can vary from person to person. This is culturally learned behaviour and often differs depending on the culture, the situation and the closeness of the relationship. If you position yourself too close to the individual, this could make the person feel anxious and uncomfortable. Likewise, if you position yourself too far away this could make the person feel isolated. When thinking about how close you should sit to a person it is important to consider their cultural beliefs and values. Personal space is a very important aspect of care work and each person is different in their acceptance of this invasion.

Key terms

Proximity relates to the distance that is maintained between people throughout the process of communication.

Touch

Touch is a very powerful means of non-verbal communication. We communicate a great deal through touch. Think about the messages given by the following: a firm handshake, a timid tap on the shoulder, a warm bear hug, a reassuring pat on the back, a patronising pat on the head, or a controlling grip on your arm.

Touch is an essential component of caring for individuals who are living with a life limiting illness, and this can take the form of holding a hand, placing a hand on a shoulder or a hug. The use of touch can be reassuring and a way of demonstrating that you care. Care must be taken though as not every person will respond in the same way to touch. If you do use touch, it is important to ensure it is well received by the other person, as some people may feel uncomfortable being touched by other people. It is also important to be aware of the importance of

appropriate timing in relation to the use of touch. For example, if an individual is struggling with difficult decisions, the use of touch may cause the person to withdraw rather than staying with the feeling they might be trying to express.

Gestures

Gestures refer to the hand and head movements or signals which many people use to emphasise what they are saying. Gestures may also help you to understand what a person is trying to communicate. There are certain common gestures that most people will automatically recognise. For example, a wave of the hand can signify hello or goodbye and thumbs up can mean all is well. Demonstrating an action may help people to understand when they find verbal communication difficult to follow. Equally a gesture such as nodding your head can indicate to a person that you are listening. Although gestures can convey meaning it is important to realise that the meaning of gestures can be very different across cultures and regions. It is therefore important to be careful to avoid misinterpretation.

Key terms

Gestures refer to the hand and head movements or signals which many people use to emphasise what they are saying.

Posture

Posture refers to the way in which you stand or sit. Your posture can indicate your confidence, openness and attitude. There are certain postures which can convey a negative attitude. For example folded arms or crossed legs can send the message that you are being defensive or are not interested in what is happening. A slouched posture may convey fatigue, poor health or low self-esteem. By contrast, a relaxed but straight posture is more likely to convey health, vitality and confidence.

Visual aids

Visual aids can be extremely useful when an individual finds verbal communication difficult. This could be because the person has little or no speech. Flash cards with pictures on are an excellent example of a visual aid.

Evidence activity

3.1 **Explain the principles of effective listening and information giving, including the importance of picking up on cues and non-verbal communication**

Explain the principles of effective listening and giving information when communicating with a person who is receiving end of life care. Why is it important to pick up on cues and non-verbal communication?

Evidence activity

3.2 **Explain how personal experiences of death and dying may affect capacity to listen and respond appropriately**

How do you think your own personal experiences of death and dying may affect your ability to listen and respond appropriately to the concerns of a person who is facing the end of their life?

3.2 **Explain how personal experiences of death and dying may affect capacity to listen and respond appropriately**

Whilst the ability to listen and respond appropriately are essential skills when supporting individuals through their end of life care experience, it is important to realise that the capacity to listen and respond appropriately can be affected by your own personal experiences of death and dying. Healthcare professionals, and especially those who work directly with individuals who are dying, are faced with potential losses every day. What a person says may trigger feelings associated with your own personal experience. If these feelings have not been resolved, this could lead to an overwhelming surge of emotion.

If you are emotionally charged, you may have a tendency to tune out what the person is saying. The emotions that are developing below the surface can then become the centre of attention.

Good listeners try to see things from the speaker's perspective. If you listen strictly from your own perspective, you may miss out on the relevance of what is being said. In order to be able to listen and respond appropriately, attention needs to be given to the person who is speaking, not on your inner turmoil.

3.3 **Give examples of internal and external coping strategies for individuals and others when facing death and dying**

Every person will experience death and dying in their own unique way. Equally, the coping strategies that a person adopts will depend on the individual's gender, culture, age, attitude, previous experiences, level of support, stage of illness and current emotions and problems. Coping strategies are useful because they allow the person to deal with the reality of what is happening to them. Coping strategies can be divided into two categories. These are internal coping strategies and external strategies.

Key terms

Coping strategies are the overall pattern of coping responses.

Internal coping strategies may include resiliency, denial, spiritual beliefs and religious beliefs.

External coping mechanisms may come from the support offered by family and friends, spiritual or religious affiliations, organisations, counselling and holistic therapies.

Exploring the internal and external coping strategies and resources a person has available to them can be helpful in assisting with crisis situations.

Evidence activity

 3.3 **Give examples of internal and external coping strategies for individuals and others when facing death and dying**

Give four examples of internal and external coping strategies that may be used by individuals and the people around them when facing death and dying.

3.4 Explain the importance of ensuring effective channels of communication are in place with others

Good communication and interpersonal skills are essential components in delivering good quality end of life care. High quality end of life care is dependent upon a multidisciplinary team approach and inter-professional communication is essential to ensure care is co-ordinated and is delivered within the plan of care. In addition, if service users and their families are truly to be part of the process of care then it is essential that they are involved in communications regarding their care and treatment options.

Service users, staff and other adults interact and communicate with each other for a variety of different reasons within the field of end of life care. For example, people communicate in order to:

- make relationships and develop relationships
- obtain and share information
- express thoughts and ideas
- give and receive support
- express feelings, wishes, needs and preferences.

Making relationships and developing relationships

Individuals communicate to make new relationships. In end of life care settings these relationships may be with service users, visitors or colleagues. Positive verbal and non-verbal communication skills, such as being friendly, smiling and shaking hands when greeting the person, are needed to make a good first impression in a relationship. End of life care involves developing meaningful professional relationships with service users, their families or carers and colleagues, by maintaining a friendly, supportive approach, and by being interested in what other people are doing and feeling. This enables service users to feel comfortable and secure, and feel that they can trust and rely on the staff who are providing support.

Obtaining and sharing information

In addition to the service user and their family, there may be many different members of the multidisciplinary team involved in the health and social care process. Members of staff will therefore need to obtain and share information about service users with colleagues and other professionals in order to co-ordinate care and to ensure the team is fully informed and updated of any changes. Staff will also need to communicate with service users or family members about the care and support they receive, or about the kinds of services and facilities that are available in the care setting.

Expressing thoughts and ideas

Members of staff working in end of life care may need to share their thoughts about care issues or about aspects of practice with other colleagues. Effective communication skills are also needed to encourage service users to talk about what they are feeling, to say what they think or to express their needs, wishes or preferences.

Giving and receiving support

Service users and their relatives often seek reassurance from care staff as a way of developing their self-confidence. In response, care staff use praise and touch, and give time and attention as a way of rewarding a person's efforts and achievements and to reassure them. Some care settings may also use support groups, staff meetings and appraisals as ways of providing staff with support and reassurance about their work performance.

Expressing feelings, wishes, needs and preferences

Members of staff who work in the field of end of life care need to find ways of encouraging service users to express their feelings and to talk about how they wish to be treated, as well as to say what they like and dislike. People will communicate in this way if they trust, and have a secure relationship with, care staff.

Effective communication is a central part of the work that must happen when providing care for people who have been diagnosed with a life limiting illness or condition. Staff working in end of life care will therefore need to develop a range of communication skills and be able to use them effectively to carry out the various aspects of their work role. They will need to be able to communicate effectively with service users, the families of service users and their colleagues, as well as colleagues from other agencies.

Evidence activity

3.4 Explain the importance of ensuring effective channels of communication are in place with others

Explain why it is important to ensure effective channels of communication are in place between health care professionals, service users and their families within the field of end of life care.

LO4 Understand how to support those involved in end of life care situations

4.1 Describe possible emotional effects on staff working in end of life care situations

Supporting people throughout end of life care can be enormously rewarding. However, it is also important to recognise that it can equally be stressful and exhausting. Many aspects of the role can contribute to work-related stress. Many members of the health and social care team have a responsibility to provide general palliative care to people who are nearing the end of their life, and this can bring with it a number of unique demands and challenges. For example, some of the unique demands on health and social care staff may include:

- being confronted with death on a daily basis – this can lead to feelings associated with **cumulative grief**

- daily confrontation with people who are in emotional and physical pain – this can lead to feelings associated with helplessness and inadequacy, especially when suffering has not been relieved
- demanding care
- the grief and sometimes anger expressed by the family
- feelings associated with the undervaluing of their role by other team members
- feelings associated with conflict due to increased contact with other professionals, especially where differences of opinion are expressed
- stress associated with higher self-expectations.

Key terms

Cumulative grief can occur where unresolved grief from a number of bereavement experiences accumulates and causes a deep feeling of bereavement.

Evidence activity

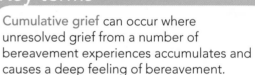

4.1 Describe possible emotional effects on staff working in end of life care situations

Outline the possible emotional effects on staff who work in end of life care environments.

Case Study

4.1 Unresolved grief

You have supported Marjorie for the last three and a half years. Over the past six months, Marjorie's health has deteriorated and she has needed more support as she has entered the end of life phase of care. You book a week's annual leave and, while you are on holiday, Marjorie dies. You never got a chance to say goodbye to her. What emotions do you think you might feel given these circumstances?

Evaluate possible sources of support for staff in end of life situations

Within a busy care setting, the feelings and needs of staff can often be overlooked. In order to prevent emotions and feelings associated with burn out and stress, it is important that staff can access support.

In the first instance it might be helpful to discuss your feelings with others within your workplace. This source of support might come from your manager or work colleagues. Your organisation may also have a dedicated pastoral service, which staff can access. Some people may also derive comfort from family and friends; however, care must be taken to ensure confidentiality is maintained.

If signs and symptoms associated with stress are causing concern specialist support may be required. Excessive or prolonged stress can lead to physical illness or problems associated with mental health. Under these circumstances support should be sought from your General Practitioner (GP). Your GP should be able to refer you for specialist support if required, for example, a therapist trained in stress management or a grief counsellor.

Evidence activity

4.2 Evaluate possible sources of support for staff in end of life care situations

Outline the sources of support for staff who work in end of life care situations.

 ## Identify areas in group care situations where others may need support in end of life care situations

If a person dies in a group setting such as a care home, careful thought and consideration must be given as to how other service users can be supported. As well as providing support for the loved ones of the deceased, there may be times when other service users will require your support. There may be times when individuals form strong bonds and friendships, and these people may need support to get through what might be a very difficult time for them.

The same could be said for married couples who are being cared for within a group setting, such as a care home. These people may have been married for many years. If one of the couple dies, this could be devastating for the bereaved partner. They may have never spent time apart in all of their years of marriage.

Evidence activity

4.3 Identify areas in group care situations where others may need support in end of life care situations

Think about your area of work and identify situations when others may need support in end of life care situations.

 ## Outline sources of emotional support for others in end of life care situations

Although the death of a loved one can be devastating, it is something that most people eventually learn to live with. For those who require additional support, it is important that they receive reassurance that help is available. Emotional support may initially be offered by care staff within the area of end of life care. However, there may be times when outside professional support may need to be accessed. Some people may find it helpful to meet and talk with other people who have been through a similar experience. Other people may benefit from seeing a bereavement counsellor. Your organisation should have a list of people who could be contacted if emotional support is required in an end of life care situation.

Evidence activity

4.4 Outline sources of emotional support for others in end of life care situations

Using any resources available to you make a resource which details the sources of support an individual could access in an end of life care situation.

LO5 Understand how symptoms might be identified in end of life care

 Identify a range of symptoms that may be related to an individual's condition, pre-existing conditions or treatment itself

Symptom control and symptom management are an essential part of end of life care. The following symptoms are among those most commonly seen in end of life care. Some of these symptoms are related to the person's condition, and others may be side effects of treatment:

- pain
- weakness and fatigue
- breathlessness (dyspnoea)
- thirst
- nausea and vomiting
- constipation
- diarrhoea
- incontinence
- fever
- mouth problems, e.g. mouth ulcers and fungal infections
- hiccups
- skin irritations
- difficulty swallowing
- restlessness and confusion
- excessive sweating
- itching
- depression
- jaundice
- insomnia
- anxiety
- confusion
- anorexia.

Evidence activity

5.1 Identify the symptoms that may be related to an individual's condition and/or treatment

Think about a service user who has been diagnosed with a life-limiting illness and make a note of all the symptoms the individual has experienced, or is experiencing.

5.2 Describe how symptoms can cause an individual and others distress and discomfort

Managing symptoms is an important part of end of life care, and it is important to remember that every person will experience different symptoms depending on their condition and the treatment they are receiving. If left untreated, the symptoms identified above could cause an individual distress and discomfort. When we are healthy, we tend to take basic activities of living such as drinking, eating, swallowing and talking for granted. However, imagine if you had a mouthful of ulcers. This could affect your ability to eat and drink and, to some extent, your ability to talk. This could be very distressing for the individual and their loved ones.

In order to effectively manage symptoms, it is important to establish the underlying cause. It should never be assumed that the symptoms are caused by the individual's primary condition. It is, however, not always easy to establish the underlying cause, as there could sometimes be a number of possible causes. Some of these may include:

- the disease or condition itself
- side effects of treatment, e.g. chemotherapy or radiotherapy
- an existing disorder, e.g. anaemia, asthma or diabetes
- environmental issues
- psychological conditions such as anxiety or depression.

Understanding the underlying causes of symptoms will have an impact on the delivery of care. It is important to realise that the failure to recognise underlying causes will contribute to on-going and worsening distress and suffering.

Evidence activity

 5.2 Describe how symptoms can cause an individual distress and discomfort

Think about a service user for whom you have been involved in delivering end of life care. Consider the symptoms the individual has experienced and describe how these symptoms have caused distress and discomfort for the individual.

5.3 Describe signs of approaching death

As a person nears death, several physical changes will occur as the body prepares for death. Although physical decline is highly individual, there are some common signs that death is approaching.

- **Loss of appetite** – During the final days the person will commonly experience anorexia. This is a sign that life is drawing to a close. At this stage the temptation to force fluid and food on the person must be avoided.
- **Changes in body temperature** – As the dying person's circulation slows down, the body temperature will drop. The skin will feel cool to the touch and may also feel clammy or damp. The lips and skin will look very pale.
- **Increased sleepiness and loss of consciousness** – As the body begins to shut down, the individual will sleep more and communicate less.

- **Loss of ability to swallow** – As the person gets weaker the ability to swallow will become more difficult.
- **Bowel and bladder weakness** – As the muscles weaken, the ability to control the bowel and bladder will deteriorate. This may lead to the person becoming incontinent and could also lead to bloating of the abdomen.
- **Decreased urine output** – Urine output will diminish as the person's intake of fluid decreases. Urine output may even cease altogether in the last 24 to 48 hours.
- **Changes in breathing** – Respiration will become slow and may become laboured. The dying person's breathing pattern may become irregular with periods of shallow and deep breaths alternating over short periods of time. Breathing may be noisy and gurgling may be heard in the back of the throat as mucous settles there.
- **Declining levels of perception and lucidity** – As death approaches the dying person may lose touch with reality. Some people also experience hallucinations. Family members may be unrecognisable to the individual and the person may not recognise his or her surroundings.
- **Agitation** – some people may experience what is known as terminal agitation. This aspect of agitation is usually treatable and it is important to monitor and ensure the person's symptoms are controlled. It is also important to ensure a peaceful environment.
- **Decline of senses** – The dying person's vision and other senses will start to deteriorate.

In order to play an effective part in symptom management, it is important to:

- Observe the person for any changes in condition or unusual signs and symptoms
- Understand some of the underlying causes of symptoms
- Appreciate the factors that can alleviate or exacerbate symptoms
- Provide support and reassurance
- Provide any therapy you are trained to deliver
- Report and accurately document your findings and actions.

Evidence activity

 Describe signs of approaching death
5.3

Describe the signs that might indicate to you that a person is approaching death.

5.4 Identify different techniques for relieving symptoms

One of the aims of end of life care is to prevent or relieve any distress a person may be experiencing. The manifestation of distress and its causes will vary from person to person. Distress can be physical or emotional, and can be related directly to the psychological aspects of living with a life-limiting condition, or to the physical symptoms that can occur as a person is nearing the end of their life.

When a person has numerous symptoms, it is important to work with them to establish which symptom needs to be addressed first.

Evidence activity

5.4 **Identify different techniques for relieving symptoms**

Think about the symptoms you have identified within Evidence activity 5.2 and identify how these symptoms are being relieved.

LO6 Understand advance care planning

6.1 Explain the difference between a care or support plan, and an advance care plan

Every person requiring support from care services will have a care plan (sometimes known as a support plan). When an individual begins to receive support, whether in hospital, in a care home, or in the community, an assessment of their day-to-day needs must be completed. Depending on the care setting, the assessment is usually completed by a nurse, senior carer or social worker, with input from other professionals, for example, physiotherapists, occupational therapists, speech and language therapists and doctors. If support involves the input of other care services, a representative of the appropriate agency that will offer support must also be involved in the assessment, so that they can be sure the agency is able to meet the individual's needs. The assessment must also involve the individual and their family and friends. When this assessment has been completed, it will form the basis for the person's care plan.

A care plan should cover every aspect of the individual's daily life. The purpose of a care plan is to provide a detailed written record of the individual's needs and wishes and identify the level of support required to meet the individual's health, personal and social care needs. Care plans should cover aspects such as: mobility, continence, washing and dressing, dietary requirements, social activities, communication and health requirements.

Risk assessments must also be included in the care plan. This is important to ensure there is a balance between keeping the individual safe and maintaining their independence. For example, a risk assessment may detail that an individual may be left unsupervised while in the bath.

In contrast to care planning, advance care planning has been defined within the guidance 'Capacity, Care Planning and Advance Care Planning in Life Limiting Illness. A Guide for Health and Social Care Staff' 2011 as:

> 'a voluntary process of discussion and review to help an individual who has capacity to anticipate how their condition may affect them in the future and, if they wish, set on record: choices about their care and treatment and / or an advance decision to refuse a treatment in specific circumstances, so that these can be referred to by those responsible for their care or treatment (whether professional staff or family carers) in the event that they lose capacity to decide once their illness progresses'.

http://www.endoflifecareforadults.nhs.uk/assets/
downloads/ACP_booklet_2011_Final_1.pdf

We can therefore assume that advance care planning is a process that is used to discuss and plan ahead. It involves the discussion and documentation of service users' wishes. Family members and friends can be involved if the service user wishes.

Advance care planning centres on discussions with a person who has capacity to make decisions about their future care and treatment. If the

Client name:		Date of birth:			Room No:	
Signatures: Client:				Key worker:		
Please tick areas to be covered by care plan:						
Continence		Medication		Washing/bathing		Mobility
Social activities		Behaviour		Diet		Dressing
Communication		Other				
Client needs, abilities and wishes				Action/support required		

Care plan for ....

Date admitted ....

Room number ....

Date of birth ....

Next of kin ....

Figure 1.7 Care plans

individual wishes, their family and friends may be included. It is recommended with the individual's agreement that discussions are documented, regularly reviewed, and communicated to key persons involved in their care.

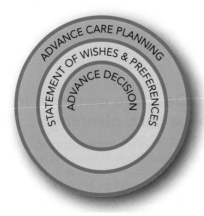

Figure 1.8 Advance care planning

The types of wishes and preferences that are commonly discussed include:

- where the individual would like to be cared for towards the end of their life – this is supported through the Preferred Priorities for Care (PPC)
- choices about the type of treatment and care they wish to receive
- choices about the type of treatment and care they would not wish to receive
- arrangements in relation to the individual's funeral.

There are two specific areas within advance care planning. These are:

1. **Advance statement of wishes and preferences** – this relates to the formalisation of what service users wish to happen to them in the future. It involves a discussion surrounding the individual's preferences, wishes and plans for their future treatment and care. This is not legally binding but can be very useful when determining a person's best interests if they lose the capacity to make decisions in the future.

2. **Advance decisions** – this clarifies what service users do not wish to happen to them in the future. The Mental Capacity Act (2005) gives people in England and Wales a statutory right to refuse treatment, through an 'advance decision'. An advance decision therefore allows service users to state what forms of treatment they wish to refuse should they become unable to decide for themselves in the future. An assessment of the individual's capacity to make that decision at that time must be undertaken, and the advance decision must be accurately formulated in order to make the advance decision legally binding. Chapter 9 of the Mental Capacity Act (MCA) 2005 Code of Practice refers specifically to advance decisions to refuse treatment.

Under the Mental Capacity Act (2005) the person making the advance decision can also appoint a lasting power of attorney (LPA) to look after their personal welfare. The lasting power of attorney is a nominated person who can make decisions about future medical treatment on behalf of the individual once the person loses the capacity to make the decision. Once an advance care plan has been drawn up, it is essential that it is reviewed on a regular basis, in order to identify any changes in wishes.

The difference between care planning and advance care planning is that the process of advance care planning can only take place when a person has the capacity to make decisions about their care in anticipation of future deterioration of their condition, which may lead to the inability to make informed decisions or communicate their wishes to others. The process of care planning comprises the care of people who may or may not have the capacity to make their own decisions. It involves a process of assessment and person-centred discussion to establish the person's needs, preferences and goals of care. It also involves making decisions about how to meet these in the context of available resources.

 ## Identify where to find additional information about advance care planning

There are many resources which provide additional information about advance care planning. Some of these are aimed at health and social care professionals and some are written in terms which are easy for service users to understand.

Additional information may come from:

- professional journals or textbooks
- formal training sessions and courses run by health and social care professionals
- informal training sessions and discussions with other members of staff who have specialist knowledge about the process of advance care planning
- reputable web links, such as those mentioned at the end of this chapter
- accredited e-learning courses such as **http://www.e-lfh.org.uk/projects/e-elca/index.html**
- your organisational policy.

Evidence activity

6.2 Identify where to find additional information about advance care planning

Make a booklet to identify all available resources that provide additional information about advance care planning. You may want to include resources aimed at health and social care staff and resources aimed at service users.

Evidence activity

6.1 Explain the difference between a care or support plan, and an advance care plan

Design a leaflet which will assist your service users' understanding of the difference between a care plan and an advance care plan.

6.3 Describe own role in advance care planning

Your role in advance care planning will depend on the organisation in which you work and your level of knowledge, experience and skill. It is therefore important to be aware of the limitations of your knowledge and the circumstances under which you may need to refer the person to a more appropriately trained member of the team. In all instances, it is essential that you work within your own sphere of competence and follow your workplace policies and procedures at all times.

Evidence activity

 6.3 **Describe your own role in advance care planning**

Describe the role you play in advance care planning.

 6.4 **Explain why, with their consent, it is important to pass on information about the individual's wishes, needs, and preferences for their end of life care**

The wishes of people approaching the end of life are not always known by members of the wider healthcare team or the service users' family. This can lead to situations where service users are denied the care that is important to them, or in the setting where they would want to receive it. This could lead to a situation in which service users' wishes and advance decisions are not taken into consideration. It is therefore essential that any significant information relating to the individual's wishes, needs and preferences are appropriately recorded and, with the consent of the service user, passed on to appropriate members of the team.

Evidence activity

6.4 **Explain why it is important to pass on information about the individual's wishes, needs, and preferences for their end of life care**

Explain the consequences of failure to pass on information about an individual's wishes, needs and preferences for their end of life care.

Assessment summary

Your reading of this chapter and completion of the activities will have prepared you to demonstrate your learning and understanding of the principles of working in end of life care. To achieve this unit, your assessor will require you to:

Learning outcomes	Assessment criteria
Learning outcome **1**: Understand current approaches to end of life care by:	(1.1) analysing the impact of national and local drivers on current approaches to end of life care See Evidence activity 1.1, p.4.
	(1.2) evaluating how a range of tools for end of life care can support the individual and others See Evidence activity 1.2, p.5.
	(1.3) analysing the stages of the local end of life care pathway See Evidence activity 1.3, p.7
Learning outcome **2**: Understand an individual's response to their anticipated death by:	(2.1) evaluating models of loss and grief See Evidence activity 2.1, p.9.
	(2.2) describing how to support the individual throughout each stage of grief See Evidence activity 2.2, p.9
	(2.3) explaining the need to explore with each individual their own specific areas of concern as they face death See Evidence activity 2.3, p.11
	(2.4) describing how an individual's awareness of spirituality may change as they approach end of life See Evidence activity 2.4, p.11
Learning outcome **3**: Understand factors regarding communication for those involved in end of life care by:	(3.1) explaining the principles of effective listening and information giving, including the importance of picking up on cues and non-verbal communication See Evidence activity 3.1, p.16
	(3.2) explaining how personal experiences of death and dying may affect capacity to listen and respond appropriately See Evidence activity 3.2, p.16

Learning outcomes	Assessment criteria	
	(3.3)	giving examples of internal and external coping strategies for individuals and others when facing death and dying See Evidence activity 3.3, p.17
	(3.4)	explaining the importance of ensuring effective channels of communication are in place with others See Evidence activity 3.4, p.18
Learning outcome **4**: Understand how to support those involved in end of life care situations by:	(4.1)	describing possible emotional effects on staff working in end of life care situations See Evidence activity 4.1, p.18
	(4.2)	evaluating possible sources of support for staff in end of life situations See Evidence activity 4.2, p.19
	(4.3)	identifying areas in group care situations where others may need support in end of life care situations See Evidence activity 4.3, p.19
	(4.4)	outline sources of emotional support for others in end of life care situations See Evidence activity 4.4, p.19
Learning outcome **5**: Understand how symptoms might be identified in end of life care by:	(5.1)	identifying a range of symptoms that may be related to an individual's condition, pre-existing conditions and treatment itself See Evidence activity 5.1, p.20
	(5.2)	describing how symptoms can cause an individual and others distress and discomfort See Evidence activity 5.2, p.21
	(5.3)	describing signs of approaching death See Evidence activity 5.3, p.22
	(5.4)	identifying different techniques for relieving symptoms See Evidence activity 5.4, p.22

Learning outcomes	Assessment criteria
Learning outcome **6**: Understand advance care planning by:	**(6.1)** explaining the difference between a care or support plan and an advance care plan See Evidence activity 6.1, p.24
	(6.2) identifying where to find additional information about advance care planning See Evidence activity 6.2, p.24
	(6.3) describing own role in advance care planning See Evidence activity 6.3, p.25
	(6.4) explaining why, with their consent, it is important to pass on information about the individual's wishes, needs, and preferences for their end of life care See Evidence activity 6.4, p.25

Good luck!

Web links

Cruse Bereavement Care	www.crusebereavementcare.org.uk
Department of Health	www.dh.gov.uk
National Council for Palliative Care	www.ncpc.org.uk
National End of Life Care Programme	www.endoflifecareforadults.nhs.uk
E-Learning for Healthcare	www.e-lfh.org.uk/projects/e-elca/index.html

For Unit EOL 302
Managing symptoms in end of life care

2

What are you finding out?

An early assessment of an individual's needs and wishes as they approach the end of life is vital to establish their preferences and choices and identify any areas of unmet need. It is important to explore the physical, psychological, social, spiritual, cultural and, where appropriate, environmental needs and/or wishes of each individual.

Managing symptoms, including pain, is an important part of end of life care. Each person will have different symptoms depending on their condition and the kind of treatment they may be having. Good management of symptoms in the final phase is one of the main concerns of people and their families. The physical comfort of dying patients requires thorough assessment, clear communication and careful prescribing.

The reading and activities in this chapter will help you to:

- Understand the effects of symptoms in relation to the delivery of care

- Understand symptoms that identify the last few days of life may be approaching

- Understand the therapeutic options available to a person.

LO1 Understand the effects of symptoms in relation to end of life care

 Identify a range of conditions where you might provide end of life care

Around 500,000 people die in England each year. The vast majority (around 99 per cent) of deaths occur in adults over the age of 18 years, and most occur in people over 65 years. The majority of deaths occur following a period of chronic illness related to conditions such as heart disease, liver disease, renal disease, diabetes, cancer, stroke, chronic respiratory disease, neurological diseases and dementia **(http://www.endoflifecarefo-radults.nhs.uk/assets/downloads/pubs_EoLC_Strategy_1.pdf)**.

'End of life care' is for anyone with an advanced progressive illness, for example, people living with cancer or cardiovascular disease, neurological conditions and many more.

This care includes the management of pain and other symptoms at the end of life, as well as psychological, social and spiritual support to help achieve the best quality end of life care for patients and their families.

 Time to reflect

1.1 Conditions requiring care at end of life

Do you know much about the conditions discussed? Are there others you know about?

Changes occur as a person's illness progresses because of the impact of the illness on the body's ability to function normally. Doctors and nurses monitor the person's physical condition and symptoms to see how they are affecting the person's wellbeing.

It is very hard to predict how long a person has to live and exactly when they will die because life expectancies vary from one person to the next. It also depends on the type of illness and the person's response to it.

Health professionals are cautious about saying when they think someone will die. Over time, they should have a clearer idea of how long the person has to live, although they can never be exact. Indicators that they will look to include:

- The impact that symptoms are having on a person's well-being
- Increasing weakness of muscles and dependency on others
- Loss of appetite and inability to swallow tablets
- Levels of consciousness.

The age profile of people at the time of death and the relative frequency of different causes of death has changed radically since the start of the past century, when infectious diseases were the major killers in this country.

Evidence activity

1.1 Signs and symptoms of liver disease

A person has been admitted to your setting with liver disease. What signs and symptoms might be present?

1.2 Identify common symptoms associated with end of life care

It is now recognised that a person has needs beyond their physical care; therefore it is important that the whole care needs of the person are met. Care should be planned to take into consideration the religious, spiritual, psychological, social and cultural as well as physical needs. This means looking at an individual as a whole person, rather than just focusing on their medical condition.

 Time to reflect

1.2 Discussing your personal wishes and preferences

How would you feel about discussing your personal wishes and preferences?

It is important that you are aware of the services that are available and that you know when these services should be accessed. The appropriate professional will assess the person's needs, and ensure appropriate care is put in place. The team will take a holistic approach to care, which means they will take into account all aspects of the service user's well-being, including their:

- physical symptoms – e.g. pain, nausea, vomiting, difficulties with eating and drinking, constipation and breathlessness
- psychological symptoms – e.g. anxiety or fear
- spiritual issues – e.g. examining feelings and considering questions such as 'Why is this happening to me?' and 'What will happen after I die?'
- social issues – e.g. looking at the best place to support the person, whether this be at home or in a care home, and also considering practical issues such as deciding where the person wishes to die.

Research and investigate

1.2 The provision of additional support for end of life care in your setting

Who are the staff in your setting who provide additional support for end of life care?

Within your healthcare environment there should be members of staff with experience and training in looking after people who are nearing end of life, and can advise other members of staff in the support of these people. In nursing homes, there should be nursing staff with appropriate skills in palliative and end of life care. All care staff should receive some training in looking after people who are dying and be aware of their physical, spiritual and emotional needs, in order to facilitate a holistic approach to care. It is vital that care staff should also only act within their level of competence, and should know when and how to call upon other members of the team for support.

Evidence activity

1.2 Jemima

Jemima has just been admitted to your setting. Draw up a plan detailing the approaches you will use to find out about her holistic needs and identify the areas you will ask about.

1.3 Explain how symptoms can cause an individual distress and discomfort

Types of pain that constitute total pain include:

- **Physical pain** – this can be caused by disease, injury or psychological stress factors. Severity will vary.
- **Emotional or psychological pain** – fear is the emotional pain most people associate with the stress of facing one's own death. However, the issues faced can also lead to depression, anxiety or guilt.
- **Social pain** – news that an individual is dying may have a great impact socially. Isolation and loneliness may result as the person's condition deteriorates and they lose social contacts.
- **Spiritual pain** – people may lose hope and not be able to make sense of what is happening. They may have difficulty finding a purpose to life. These factors may cause great pain.
- **Religious pain** – a dying person may feel as if they have been deserted by God or are being punished. Lack of access to places of worship and ministers of religion and being unable to carry out religious rituals may also increase pain.
- **Cultural pain** – people may feel cut off from their culture and community or country. They may experience a language barrier, which means they cannot always make their needs and wishes known. Some individuals may become distressed by others' lack of understanding and respect for cultural issues such as ritual, customs, traditions or dietary requirements.

All types of pain should be viewed as a whole. Treating physical pain is obviously a priority, as this may in itself cause emotional pain. However, it must also be recognised that other types of pain can increase or aggravate physical pain – therefore, treatment for other types of pain can contribute to the relief of physical pain.

Evidence activity

1.3 Finding out about complementary therapies

A person says they do not know anything about complementary therapies. How can you help them find out more about them?

1.4 Evaluate the significance of the individual's own perception of their symptoms

The strong emotions experienced by people receiving personal care

Individuals who have a life-limiting illness and who are unable to independently meet their personal care needs will have these needs met as part of the palliative care package. An individual not only has to come to terms with their life-limiting illness, but also, as their condition deteriorates, with the need for assistance with personal care.

Having to rely on others to meet personal care needs, which are private, can provoke strong emotions. Therefore, as a healthcare worker you will have to support the individual to come to terms with their loss of independence and to understand the emotions experienced in having their personal care needs met.

Emotions experienced may include:

- **Fear** – the individual may fear the unknown, losing their independence or losing control over their life and body. They may also be afraid of experiencing pain while personal care needs are being met. Individuals may fear the healthcare staff that will assist them, be afraid the healthcare staff will forget about them, or not meet their needs in a satisfactory manner. Also, new and unfamiliar aids or equipment can provoke fear in some people.

- **Feeling violated** – going to the toilet, washing and bathing are private matters and having to rely on strangers to meet these needs can lead some people to feel violated. A person who has been abused or who is painfully shy may feel violated when washed in intimate areas, or they may feel vulnerable, or feel as though they are being abused.

- **Helplessness** – being reliant on others to meet your personal care needs can provoke feelings of helplessness. As their health deteriorates and the individuals become more dependent, they may experience feelings of helplessness because they have to rely on others to meet their needs.

- **Loss of identity** – many people feel that in losing their independence and becoming reliant on others, they are not the person they used to be and they are unsure of their identity and their station in life. This can lead to lower self-esteem and a lower sense of self-worth.

- **Embarrassment and humiliation** – having to rely on others to meet your needs can be embarrassing and humiliating, especially when being assisted to use the toilet or wash intimate parts of your body. Some individuals also find it embarrassing to even have to ask for support, regardless of the type of assistance required.

Research and investigate

1.4 What approaches can you think of to reassure a person?

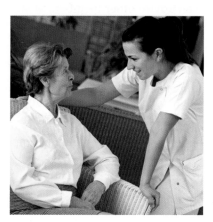

Figure 2.1 Personal care

Promoting positive emotions

As a healthcare worker assisting individuals to meet personal care needs, you can promote positive emotions in the following ways.

- Treat the individual holistically, taking into consideration their physical, spiritual, psychological and social needs, not just concentrating on their illness.
- Involve the individual in care planning and review of care plans. With the individual's permission, family and other carers should be involved in the planning and delivery of care.
- Acknowledge and validate the individual's feelings.
- Promote independence and choice whenever possible; however, do not set the individual up to fail.
- Maintain the individual's privacy and dignity at all times.
- Value and respect the individual as a person, as well as their feelings, thoughts and opinions.
- Ensure you are familiar with and confident in your ability to use any aids or equipment the individual needs.
- Ensure you follow care plans and risk assessments when providing personal care.
- Check with the individual on the level of assistance they require, as their needs may fluctuate depending on their illness.
- Use time, when meeting personal care needs, to chat and build up a relationship. Remember to explain to the individual what you are doing, or going to do, and obtain their permission.
- Ensure you are prepared to carry out personal care activities; e.g. you have the toiletries ready, the bathroom has been prepared, the individual's choice of clothing has been laid out in readiness and any equipment or aids are to hand.

Evidence activity

 Effective pain management and review

Prepare a list of actions you would need to take to ensure all aspects of pain management were effective and reviewed regularly.

LO2 Be able to manage symptoms of end of life care

2.1 Demonstrate a range of techniques to provide symptom relief

Body language and non-verbal communication aid understanding

We all need to communicate with other people. Communicating our needs, wishes and feelings is vital – not only to improve our quality of life, but also to preserve our sense of identity. Pain and discomfort has many causes and it can manifest itself as a physical, psychological or emotional problem. Signs and symptoms of pain and discomfort can be many and varied, including:

- General body tension
- Verbalising the need for analgesia (pain killers)
- Complaining of pain
- Restricted movement/reluctance to move
- Pointing to/holding the affected part
- Swelling/deformity/inflammation
- Crying or other signs of distress
- Non-verbal signs, e.g. facial expressions, posture, etc.
- Agitation/confusion/irritability/fidgeting/ nervous habits
- Sleeplessness (insomnia), disturbed sleep, restlessness
- Depression and/or anxiety
- Changes in behaviour – withdrawal or aggression
- Signs of fear or reluctance to seek medical advice – verbalising worries about ill health
- Light headedness, fainting, nausea or vomiting.

Time to reflect

2.1 Failing to meet needs and preferences and not listening properly

How would you feel if your needs and preferences were not being met and you were not being listened to properly?

It is important for healthcare staff to be aware of all aspects of verbal and non-verbal communication when communicating with individuals. An individual who is in pain may deny this verbally. However, their non-verbal communication may indicate otherwise; for example, they may grimace and flinch away from touch; also the tone of their voice may sound flat. For someone who cannot communicate verbally, non-verbal signs may be the only indication that a person is experiencing pain or discomfort.

Pain and discomfort can be alleviated using a variety of measures involving various members of the care team and other care professionals:

- Care professionals and care workers within the care team
- Nurses – specialist nurses such as Macmillan Nurses
- Doctors (GPs, physicians, surgeons, pain control specialists)
- Managers
- Physiotherapists will treat people following an operation, injury or stroke, using a combination of exercise and aids and equipment
- Chiropodist – will treat foot and nail problems which will relieve pain and discomfort for individuals, especially when walking or standing
- Dentist – to treat toothache, gum disease, neuralgia and infections (abscesses, etc.)
- Occupational therapists – can provide aids and equipment to increase independence and maximise the individual's comfort
- Counsellors.

Medication

Over the counter medication does not require a prescription, and can be purchased from a variety of shops or a local pharmacy. Paracetamol, aspirin or ibuprofen can be purchased under a number of trade names for pain relief. Items such as cod-liver oil capsules (to help individuals suffering from arthritis), laxatives (for constipation) or antihistamines (for hay fever) can also be purchased.

Although a pharmacist will give individuals advice on safe use, generally we read the instructions and recommendations on the packet or bottle and use our own judgement for use.

Allopathic medication

This is orthodox medical treatment using drugs that treat and alleviate specific symptoms and disease. The medication, prescribed by a GP or other qualified practitioner such as a dentist or nurse, is obtained from the pharmacy and administered at times, and in doses, specified by the pharmacist. Medication would include:

- Analgesia – painkillers, e.g. morphine
- Laxatives – to relieve constipation
- Antihistamines – to relieve symptoms of allergies
- Anti-inflammatory – to treat arthritis and joint pain
- Antacids – to relieve symptoms caused by digestive problems
- Antibiotics – to treat infections
- Antidepressants and anxiolytics – to relieve anxiety and depression.

Medication administration

It is important that you recognise your role in the administration, monitoring and storage of medication. It is vital that medication is handled, stored and administered safely. It is suggested that you, as a care worker, undertake a recognised educational course to ensure you understand how to deal with medication safely. This is particularly relevant to care workers who are involved in the administration of medication within their care environment.

Group of drugs designed to relieve pain

An important aspect of end of life care is the relief of pain and control of symptoms. This may be achieved through the use of drugs. In order to be able to support the individual and the doctors and nurses trained in pain management, it is important that healthcare workers are not only familiar with their workplace policies and procedures, but also have an understanding of the methods and issues relating to pain and symptom control.

It is important for you as a healthcare worker to undertake suitable and appropriate training relating to the storing, recording, administering or disposal of medication to ensure that you know and understand how to manage it safely.

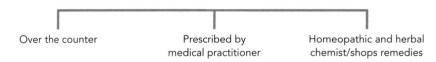

Over the counter Prescribed by medical practitioner Homeopathic and herbal chemist/shops remedies

Figure 2.2 Medication can be obtained in a number of ways

> **Homeopathic medicine** – this refers to herbal remedies or alternative or non-conventional therapies such as hypnotherapy, acupuncture, vitamins or cesium.
>
> **Allopathic medicine** – many medical dictionaries define the term allopathic medicine as the treatment of disease using conventional medical therapies, as opposed to the use of alternative medical or non-conventional therapies.
>
> Examples of allopathic medicine include anti-cancer medicines, antidepressant medicines or physiotherapy.
>
> http://www.bio-medicine.org/medicine-definition/Allopathic_medicine/

The Medicines Act (1968) was the first comprehensive legislation on medicines in the UK. Together with any additional statutory legislation, it provides the legal framework for the manufacture, licensing, prescription, supply and administration of medicines. The Act classifies medicines into the following categories:

- **Prescription-only medicines (POMs)** – these are medicines that may be supplied or administered to a patient only on the instruction of an appropriate practitioner or a trained person who is listed as a nurse prescriber.
- **Pharmacy-only medicines (Ps)** – these can be purchased from a registered primary care pharmacy, provided that the pharmacist supervises the sale.
- **General sale list medicines (GSLs)** – these need neither a prescription, nor the supervision of a pharmacist and can be obtained from retail outlets. Generally, no medication should be administered without a prescription. However, local policies or patient group directions may have been developed to allow the limited administration of medicines in this group to meet the needs of the patient.

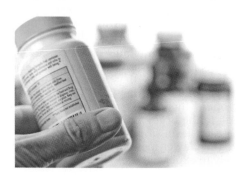

Figure 2.3 Pain relief

As well as being classified as POMs, Ps or GSLs, medicines can be classified according to the physical effects they have on the human system; for example, analgesics are a class of drugs used to relieve pain. The pain relief induced by analgesics occurs either by blocking pain signals going to the brain, or by interfering with the brain's interpretation of the signals, without producing anaesthesia or loss.

Importance of planning activities around analgesia

It is important for healthcare staff to have a knowledge and understanding of which activities cause or may cause the individual pain. This will then enable healthcare staff to plan for these activities to take place after analgesia medication has been administered and taken effect. For example, an individual who experiences severe pain in the mornings should not be assisted to wash and dress until their analgesia has been administered and has started to take effect.

Any activity may cause pain to an individual, so it is important for healthcare staff to assess which activities cause pain before developing the individual's care plan.

World Health Organisation's (WHO) 'Analgesic Ladder'

WHO has developed a three-step 'ladder' (model) for cancer pain relief. If pain occurs, there should be prompt oral administration of drugs in the following order: non-opioids (aspirin and paracetamol); then, as necessary, mild opioids (codeine); then strong opioids such as morphine, until the patient is free of pain. To calm fears and anxiety, additional drugs – 'adjuvants' – should be used. To maintain freedom from pain, drugs should be given 'by the clock', that is every three to six hours, rather than 'on demand'. This three-step approach of administering the right drug in the right dose at the right time is inexpensive and 80 to 90 per cent effective. Surgical intervention on appropriate nerves may provide further pain relief if drugs are not wholly effective.

Key terms

The World Health Organisation (WHO) is the directing and coordinating authority for health within the United Nations system. It is responsible for providing leadership on global health matters, shaping the health research agenda, setting norms and standards, articulating evidence-based policy options, providing technical support to countries and monitoring and assessing health trends.

Time to reflect

2.1 Your experience of using complementary therapies

Have you had any experience of using complementary therapies? If so which therapy did you use and what impact did it have?

Complementary therapy, alternative therapy and integrated medicine

What is the difference between complementary and alternative medicine?

The terms 'complementary medicine' and 'alternative medicine' often are used interchangeably, but the two are different. Complementary therapies are used together with traditional western medicine. For example, you may take opioids to manage your day-to-day pain and use guided imagery to help manage a breakthrough pain episode. Alternative medicine is used in place of conventional medicine. For example, using a special diet to treat your arthritis instead of using medications recommended by a doctor is using alternative medicine.

Complementary techniques to manage pain include diet, exercise, biofeedback, massage, chiropractic care, acupuncture, and self-regulation techniques such as self-hypnosis, relaxation training, yoga, reiki (a natural healing process using the hands to tap a universal life energy) and Jin Shin Jyutsu (a process to balance the body's energies to bring optimal health and well-being).

'Integrated medicine (or integrative medicine as it is referred to in the United States) is practising medicine in a way that selectively incorporates elements of complementary and alternative medicine into comprehensive treatment plans' alongside traditional methods of diagnosis and treatment. Integrated medicine focuses 'on health and healing rather than disease and treatment', viewing individuals 'as whole people with minds and spirits' **(http://www.bmj.com/cgi/content/extract/322/7279/119?ck=nck)**.

Research and investigate

2.1 Find out about gate control theory

What is the gate control theory?

Gate control theory

The way in which we experience pain is very complex. All sorts of factors influence our experience, including our thoughts and feelings. For example, you will probably be aware that there are times when, even though you have pain, you are only dimly aware of it. This can happen, for example, when you are really engrossed in doing something interesting or having to face a situation that demands all your attention. A very good example of this are the stories you might have heard about wounded soldiers, who despite being seriously injured will continue in battle and not really be aware of much pain until after the danger has passed.

On the other hand, you will probably be aware of how in some circumstances your pain can feel much worse. Indeed, you may find that the more you think about your pain, the worse it can feel. Nerves from all over the body run to the spinal cord, which is the first main meeting point for the nervous system. In the spinal cord, you might imagine a series of gates into which messages about pain arrive from all over the body.

These gates can sometimes be much more open than at other times. This is important because it is through these gates that messages from your body pass towards your brain. If the gates are more open, then a lot of pain messages pass through to the brain and you are likely to experience a high level of pain. If the gates are more closed, then fewer messages get through and you are likely to experience less pain.

Examples of complementary or alternative therapies include:

- **Acupuncture** – an ancient system of healing developed in China and other eastern countries. Fine needles are inserted into the body at various pressure points to relieve pain or treat a variety of conditions.
- **Acupressure (Shiatsu)** – based on the same principles as acupuncture but without the needles, concentrating on meridians or energy lines.
- **Aromatherapy** – the systematic use of essential oils in holistic treatments to improve physical well-being. Oils may be heated in a burner or massaged into the body.
- **Chiropractic therapy** – specialises in the diagnosis and treatment of conditions that are due to mechanical dysfunction of the joints and their effects on the nervous system. Chiropractors use their hands to adjust the joints of your spine and extremities where signs of restriction in movement are found, improving mobility and relieving pain.
- **Counselling** – during counselling sessions the client is encouraged to explore various aspects of their life and feelings, talking freely and openly in a way that is rarely possible with friends or family.
- **Reflexology** (sometimes called **zone therapy**) – a therapy in which the nerve endings primarily in the feet are stimulated by specific massage techniques to effect changes in another part of the body and thereby create health and help overcome disease.

It is important that the client's individual choice to use complementary or alternative therapies should be respected and planning for those therapies must be taken into account.

Evidence activity

2.1 Approaches to symptom relief

Investigate the approaches used in your work setting and find out how effective they are.

2.2 Describe own role in supporting therapeutic options used in symptom relief

It is important that carers provide support for people in the final hours of their life and every effort should be made to allow the person to express their needs and wishes and share their feelings and fears. This will include the implementation of therapeutic options for symptom relief.

Pacing and spacing activities

Pacing is a technique that a person can use to gradually increase their level of activity. If they have chronic pain, they might find that they have good days, when they can get on with things around the house or do something that they enjoy, and bad days, when they can do very little. As time goes on, some people find that they have fewer good days and more bad days. Pacing is all about breaking this pattern and gradually increasing what they can do. It should be possible to pace any activity, although in everyday life, we are not used to doing things gradually – we like to get things done quickly.

A person should start by choosing one or more activities that they want to be able to do, or be able to do for longer, for example, walking, sitting, standing, etc. If it's the first time they have tried pacing, ask then not to be too ambitious. Encourage them to choose an activity that they find more difficult, but not impossible. Set a baseline amount of time in which they can easily and comfortably achieve the activity. Then ask them to practise that activity regularly, every day if possible, on good days and bad. Then gradually build up the amount of time they spend doing this activity, but never do more than they planned. Write down the amount of time they spent on the activity on each occasion and this will help them to see how much they are improving.

Spacing involves breaking down an activity into manageable chunks and taking some time out between each chunk to rest and relax. By dividing up tasks in this way, the person can assess how they feel and how they are getting on with the task.

Goal setting

Chronic pain can affect lots of different aspects of a person's life. Individuals may find that they have had to give up going to places or doing things that they used to enjoy because they are afraid that this may make them feel worse. Also, it may be a little frightening to think about starting something new. Goal setting is rather like pacing – a person can use it to gradually build up the activities that they do. It's all about giving the person some control back, rather than letting the pain take over.

A goal is something that the person would like to achieve. It may be going to the cinema, walking the dog, or playing with their children or grandchildren. They could have all kinds of different goals, which can be either short- or long-term.

There are four golden rules for setting goals:

1. The goal must be realistic.
2. It must be something you both can measure.
3. It should be the person's own goal – don't let someone else pick it for the person.
4. The person should not be too ambitious to start with – encourage them to pick something that's important to them, but not impossible.

The first step is to decide on the goal. Then ask the person to think about all the things they need to do to achieve that goal. It might help to write this information down on a piece of paper. Say, for example, that their goal is to start driving their car again. There are lots of things involved in this:

- getting in and out of the car
- sitting in the driver's seat
- turning their head to look in the mirror
- twisting to put on their seat belt
- moving the pedals up and down
- leaning forward over the steering wheel
- pulling the handbrake on
- changing gear
- opening and closing the door
- concentrating on the road
- looking to the side as they pull out of a junction.

Now look at each of these activities in turn: what do they have problems with? If, for example, they have a problem with sitting, they should start by gradually increasing the amount of time that they sit in the driver's seat. To start with, they might only be able to sit for a minute or two, but after a few weeks, they should hopefully be able to build this up to 15 minutes, or so. They may also want to make practical changes, such as making use of back supports and wider mirrors.

It's important to review their progress regularly – about once a week if possible – and rethink some of the person's methods if they're not working. Always tell the person to remember that each small step is an achievement in itself, and that lots of small steps can help them take one big leap.

Assertiveness/communication

People with chronic pain sometimes lose their confidence, finding it hard to express their needs. If they don't express their needs clearly, this can increase their tension, which can increase their pain. So it's important for them to communicate well and to be assertive. They can be encouraged to do this by following the simple tips given below.

- Be firm and say what they mean.
- Ask them to try not to complain, plead or be apologetic.
- Don't shout or raise their voice, keep it calm and low.
- Make sure their message is clear, rather than expecting people to guess what they are getting at.
- Don't tell people what to do, but explain to them why they are asking them to do something.
- Ask for help when they need it.
- When they are asking for something, say 'I want' instead of 'I need' and 'I don't want' instead of 'I cannot'.
- Ask them to try and be precise and to the point – don't beat about the bush!

Research and investigate

 2.2 What role would a carer play in identifying a person's needs?

Stress

Stress and tension can make pain worse, so it's important that the person learns how to cope with (or even avoid) stress. This involves knowing what it is and recognising when they are suffering from it. When undertaking activities they must be sensitive to the feelings that they are having, especially in relation to any pain that they may experience. Being aware of their emotions and taking action to calm themselves down and relax, despite the pain, will require practice and patience.

There are a number of ways of coping with stress, including:

- being able to relax
- having someone to talk to and confide in
- being able to find a practical solution to the problem, rather than worrying about it
- using pacing techniques and breathing exercises.

When a person experiences acute pain, it makes them rest so that healing can take place. For example, if you sprained your wrist, the pain would stop you using it so that it can heal. However, with chronic pain, the person may feel pain even if there is no injury and no healing. This pain causes them to avoid certain movements and activities, making their muscles and joints stiff. This, in turn, makes the pain worse – this is called the pain cycle.

Coping with flare-ups

From time to time, the person may find that they experience periods of increased pain, sometimes called flare-ups. Although these flare-ups don't usually last very long, they often come on quickly and without much warning, so they can be difficult to cope with. It may be tempting for the person to go back to their old habits, such as taking more medication or going to bed. Encourage them to try not to do this. Flare-ups may happen, and if they do then all we can do is accept that. Coping with flare-ups is a skill and will grow with time and experience. They might also find that preparing in advance for any flare-ups can really reduce their distress.

Encourage the person to:

- recognise what is happening
- not panic
- take their medications regularly
- if they are unable to continue with their exercises for a couple of days, start slowly and reset their goals if they need to
- try to think positively – negative thoughts can make things worse.

Relaxation

Learning relaxation techniques can be very useful in that such skills can help individuals to cope with and manage pain. Anxiety, tension and stress can make the pain worse. Also, the pain itself can lead to anxiety, tension and stress, so it's a vicious circle. The trick is to break this cycle and relaxation can help to do this.

It sounds easy, but learning to relax takes time. It is important to practise everyday. The person must not be too ambitious when they first start – also, it's best not to try the techniques if they are having a really bad day, as they probably won't work. However, as they get better at relaxing, they will be able to use the techniques when they are having a bad day, and will even be able to practise when they are out and about, standing in a queue, sitting in the car, etc. They might find it useful to keep a relaxation diary – make a note of the type of relaxation exercise they did, when and where they did it, and how it felt. This diary should help them to see an improvement in their relaxation skills.

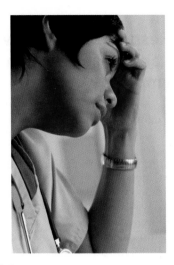

Figure 2.4 **Stress**

Sleep

Those with chronic pain often find that they have problems sleeping. They might find it difficult to get off to sleep, or find that they wake up during the night because of their pain. Unfortunately, the more they try to sleep, the harder it sometimes becomes. This can increase their stress levels, which can make the pain worse, and this, in turn, makes it more difficult to sleep. So, it's a vicious circle. If this sounds familiar, encourage the person to try following the advice given below:

- Try not to nap during the day, no matter how tired they feel – do something else instead.
- Avoid tea, coffee, alcohol and cigarettes for four hours before they go to bed.
- Wait until they feel tired before they go to bed.
- Try to go to bed at the same time each night.
- Do not read, eat or watch TV in bed.
- Make sure that their bed is comfortable – use pillows to support their legs and back.
- Use relaxation and breathing exercises in bed.
- If they can't get off to sleep, encourage them to get up and do something, such as reading or relaxation exercises.
- Get up at the same time every morning, regardless of how much they slept during the night.

Exercise

If individuals have chronic pain, they may be afraid to do exercise, but staying active, within realistic limits, can be very beneficial.

Breathing

The way that we breathe is very important when we are in pain. This may sound strange, as breathing is something we don't usually think about! However, when we are in pain, our breathing may be shallow or we may find that we are holding our breath. This can lead to tension, which may make the pain worse. The trick is to take time to think about our breathing, making sure it is slow and relaxed.

Non-medical treatment for pain

Examples of non-medical treatment for pain, in addition to analgesics and special pain medications, include:

- support and counselling:
  - psychological, spiritual and emotional support and counselling should accompany pain medications. Pain can be harder to bear when there is guilt, fear of dying, loneliness, anxiety, depression
- answering questions and explaining what is happening is important to relieve fear and anxiety
- deep breathing and relaxation techniques, unless the patient is psychotic or severely depressed
- distraction, music, imagining a calm scene.

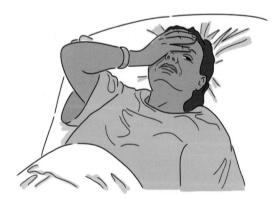

Figure 2.5 Indicators of pain

Evidence activity

2.2 Supporting therapeutic options used in symptom relief

Select two therapeutic options used in symptom relief and explain how they are used.

2.3 Respond to an individual's culture and beliefs in managing their symptoms

There are various ways in which healthcare staff are able to demonstrate that they are meeting an individual's cultural and religious beliefs, including:

- Assessing a person's religious, cultural and spiritual needs on an individual basis. The assessment may need to be reviewed periodically to meet the changing needs of the individual.
- Consulting with the individual and their family about religious, cultural and spiritual matters, including prayer, diet and routines of personal hygiene.
- Respecting and, where necessary, making arrangements for sacred practices.
- Making arrangements for priests and other religious figures to visit the individual.
- Referring the individual to a hospice/hospital chaplain, appropriate religious leader or support group that addresses spiritual issues during illness.
- Reassuring the person that the rites of their religion and culture will be fully respected after their death.

Supporting spiritual and cultural needs

There are various ways in which healthcare staff are able to demonstrate that they are meeting an individual's spiritual and cultural needs.

Spiritual needs:

- Appreciating that everyone has a spiritual dimension.
- Recognising that some people will have a religious and/or cultural element to their spirituality.
- Practising active listening and being mindful of one's non-verbal messages.
- Appreciating that people will express their spirituality and possible spiritual pain in different ways.
- Appreciating that there may be conflicts within families around spiritual issues.

Cultural needs:

- Treat each person as an individual.
- Learn from the individual and their family and ask questions about cultural beliefs and practices.
- Research the different cultural groups within the healthcare setting.
- Be sensitive to a person's past as this may affect how the individual responds and behaves.
- Provide clear information in a user friendly format.

All aspects of health and safety are covered by legislation.

The health care worker has a vital role to play in the management and control of distressing symptoms. Care workers should:

- Observe the person for any changes in condition or unusual signs or symptoms
- Provide support
- Give reassurance and whatever forms of therapy staff are trained to offer
- Report and document findings.

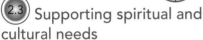

Time to reflect

(2.3) Supporting spiritual and cultural needs

Why is it important a person has their spiritual and cultural needs met?

Research and investigate

(2.4) Supporting a person effectively

If you are to support a person effectively what actions do you need to take prior to any activity?

It is important for healthcare staff to respect an individual's spiritual and cultural beliefs and practices regardless of their own beliefs. Healthcare staff should do their utmost to meet the spiritual, religious and cultural needs of individuals in their care. If healthcare staff are unable to meet these needs, help and advice should be sought from managers. Healthcare staff will also need to report to managers any discrimination or withholding of an individual's rights.

Evidence activity

(2.3) Phoebe

Phoebe is feeling very demoralised, her treatment is taking longer than expected and she is feeling very unwell. What approaches could support her and make her feel more positive?

Actively support the comfort and well being in end of life care

Mobility is important for people who have a life-limiting illness. It can help keep up morale and aid physical comfort.

Supporting a person with nausea and vomiting

Most people have, at some time in their lives, experienced nausea and or vomiting and understand how extremely unpleasant it is. These symptoms in a person who is dying may occur for a variety of reasons, such as:

- The illness itself – especially digestive tract disease
- Medication side effects – some analgesia cause this
- Constipation
- Chemotherapy
- Strong odours.

It is vital that these symptoms are controlled as soon as possible. This can be achieved in a variety of ways:

- Identify cause – it may sometimes be possible to remove the cause, e.g. a strong smell.
- Formulate a plan. Involve the person and their family.
- Use of anti-emetics – these can be used in conjunction with analgesia and can be administered orally, by injection or via a syringe driver.
- Reassure and support the person and their family. Remember you can offer practical help as well as information and emotional support.

- Clean up the vomit and the person – ensure privacy and dignity. Do this promptly.
- Ensure that the person has access to a vomit bowl, tissues and water and has a means of calling for assistance.
- Help the person to clean their mouth and brush their teeth.
- Dispose of all contaminated waste and linen appropriately.
- Clear away promptly.
- Ventilate and deodorise the room.
- Use recommended cleaning fluids.
- Use PPE (e.g. apron and gloves).
- Always offer reassurance and support. The person may be very embarrassed, and family may find the smell distressing and clearing up difficult and unpleasant.

Encourage independence when moving an individual

There are many ways in which an individual can help and cooperate with you when carrying out moving and handling procedures. It is important that this is encouraged, as cooperation from an individual is invaluable, both for maintaining their independence and for assisting those carrying out the move.

Any independence which can be achieved is also important in terms of the individual's self-esteem and sense of well-being. A person may be able to transfer themselves from a wheelchair to a chair, or into bed; this is important as a means of independence and mobility and exercise.

You may be able to use self-help techniques when an individual needs a bed pan. Rather than having to be lifted manually, they can be encouraged to bend the knees and raise their bottom to allow the bed pan to be slid underneath them.

Techniques like this require active cooperation from the individual and are obviously not suitable for use when individuals are not able to cooperate.

Where there is any conflict between the individual's wishes and health and safety issues, it is important that these are discussed and that you explain to them that you must adhere to any statutory regulations to protect you and them. Every attempt must be made to reach a compromise so that you can carry out moving and handling procedures according to the guidelines, while also still meeting the needs of the individual.

Evidence activity

2.4 Encouraging and supporting independence

Why is it important to encourage independence and how can you support this?

2.5 Recognise symptoms that identify the last few days of life may be approaching

It is notoriously difficult to predict when death will occur. Symptoms and signs of death approaching include day-by-day deterioration, gaunt appearance and profound weakness; the patient needs assistance with all care, and may be bed-bound; difficulty swallowing medicines; reduced intake of food and fluids and drowsiness or reduced cognition. The patient is often no longer able to cooperate with carers.

Traditionally, care was planned and delivered based on the medical condition and resulting physical needs of the individual. Each medical problem tended to have a generic care plan, as care plans were not tailored to meet the individual person's unique individual needs.

Within the whole person approach, or the holistic approach to care, the care plan looks beyond the physical need and will take into consideration the individual's:

- psychological or emotional needs
- cultural needs/beliefs and practices
- spiritual needs/beliefs and practices
- social needs.

Time to reflect

2.5 Compare care delivery in the past with current approaches

How was care delivered in the past? How does this differ from current approaches?

A human's needs cannot be compartmentalised, as they are all integrated and overlap. Being diagnosed with a life-limiting illness will probably have an adverse effect on all aspects of a person's life. Therefore, as a carer you will need to look at the individual as a whole and not just their medical condition. It is important to remember this throughout the individual's illness; even in the last few hours of life they will have more than just physical needs.

Everybody is different and will experience and respond to illness differently. Therefore, if care staff concentrate on the illness rather than the person behind it, they will be unable to meet the principles of palliative care.

Developing a care plan that covers the whole person makes it easier for staff to see beyond the illness to the person before they became ill. To be able to do this, the care staff will need to consider the individual's biography and identity. This information will give the staff involved in the care and support of the person an excellent background into subjects of interest, which they may discuss when communicating with that person.

Supportive care helps the patient and their family to cope with the condition and treatment of it – from pre-diagnosis, through the process of diagnosis and treatment, cure, continuing illness or death and into bereavement. It also helps the patient to maximise the benefits of treatment and to live as well as possible with the effects of the disease. It is given equal priority alongside diagnosis and treatment. Supportive care should be fully integrated with diagnosis and treatment. It encompasses:

- self-help and support
- user involvement
- information giving
- psychological support
- symptom control
- social support
- rehabilitation
- complementary therapies
- spiritual support
- end of life and bereavement care.

Evidence activity

2.5 Matthew

Matthew requires a great deal of support; his pain is severe. Who else should you consult when planning how to meet Matthew's needs?

LO3 Understand how to manage symptoms of pain

3.1 Identify signs that may indicate that an individual is experiencing pain

Not all individuals are able to express pain. Some cannot find the words to describe the pain they are experiencing. However, there are signs that indicate an individual is experiencing some form of pain. These signs may include:

- request for analgesia
- complaints of pain
- general body tension
- tense facial expression
- constant fidgeting, or nervous habits
- agitation
- anxiety
- changes in a person's behaviour, e.g. withdrawn or aggressive
- flinching away from touch
- holding/protecting painful area
- inflammation/swelling/redness
- pasty, wan complexion
- crying
- sleeplessness
- pointing to affected area.

Evidence activity

 3.1 Your understanding of pain

Explain in your own words what you think pain is.

Time to reflect

3.2 Your personal experience of pain

When you have experienced pain what made it worse, and what made it better?

 3.2 **Describe factors that can influence an individual's perception of pain**

Accurate assessment of pain is essential to plan appropriate interventions or treatments. Uncontrolled pain limits a person's ability to self-care, affects their response to illness and reduces their quality of life. In keeping with the 'Total Pain' model, assessment should consider the following domains:

- **Physical** – people may experience pain because of physical factors related to the underlying disease, e.g. cancer, abdominal distension from ascites. The pain may be related to treatment, e.g. surgery, chemotherapy, radiotherapy, drug-related neuropathies. There may also be associated factors, e.g. constipation, pressure sores, bladder spasm, stiff joints.

- **Psychosocial** – psychosocial factors may have a profound influence on an individual's perception and experience of pain and can affect how the patient responds emotionally and behaviourally. There is a large body of scientific evidence to support the role of anxiety and depression, fear, pain-related beliefs and coping styles in the mediation of pain perception in chronic non-malignant pain.

- **Spiritual** – people suffering from chronic unremitting pain can experience spiritual distress/pain. The spiritual dimension of an individual includes meaning, relatedness, hope and forgiveness – this may or may not include a religious belief system.

It is imperative that patients' anxieties and frequent misconceptions related to the above factors are explored. Pain will not be adequately controlled unless patients feel a degree of control over their situation. To ignore psychological and spiritual aspects of care may often be the reason for seemingly intractable pain. The patient, if competent and able to communicate, is the most reliable assessor of pain, and where possible should be the prime judge of their pain.

Table 2.1 Factors affecting pain tolerance in individuals

Pain tolerance is lowered by:	Pain tolerance is raised by:
• Discomfort	• Relief of symptoms
• Insomnia	• Sleep
• Fatigue	• Rest or physiotherapy
• Anxiety	• Relaxation therapy
• Fear	• Explanation/ support
• Anger	• Understanding/ empathy
• Boredom	• Diversion
• Sadness	• Listening
• Depression	• Elevation of mood
• Introversion	• Finding meaning and significance
• Social abandonment	• Social inclusion
• Mental isolation	• Support to express emotions

Evidence activity

 Difficulties facing a person experiencing increased pain

Discuss the difficulties you think might be faced by the person when experiencing increased pain.

3.3 Describe a range of assessment tools for monitoring pain in individuals, including those with cognitive impairment

Pain assessment tools

The range of pain measurement tools is vast, and includes both uni-dimensional and multi-dimensional methods.

Uni-dimensional tools:

- measure one dimension of the pain experience, e.g. intensity
- are accurate, simple, quick, easy to use and understand
- are commonly used for acute pain assessment
- have a verbal rating scale and the verbal descriptor scales, e.g. none, mild, moderate, severe; and are commonly used for postoperative pain assessment.

Multi-dimensional pain assessment tools:

- provide information about the qualitative and quantitative aspects of pain
- may be useful if neuropathic pain is suspected
- require patients to have good verbal skills and sustained concentration, as they take longer to complete than uni-dimensional tools.

Research and investigate

3.3 Describe how an assessment tool works

Choose an assessment tool and describe how it works.

Observational tools may be used with patients who are unconscious/sedated and cognitively impaired to assess physiological responses and/or behaviours, for example, facial expressions, limb movements, vocalisation, restlessness and guarding.

Global scales may be useful at the end of a pain management intervention to measure the patient's perception of the overall effectiveness of an intervention. They examine the inconvenience or unpleasantness of the intervention and the personal meaningfulness of any improvement in the patient's pain and function.

Table 2.2 Selection of uni-dimensional and multi-dimensional pain assessment tools

Uni-dimensional pain measurement tools	Multi-dimensional pain measurement tools
- Visual analogue scales - Verbal rating scales - Graphic rating scales - Verbal descriptor scales - Body diagrams - Computer graphic scales - Picture scales - Coin scales - Numerical rating scales	- McGill pain questionnaire (short and long) - Brief pain inventory (short and long) - Behavioural pain scales - Pain/comfort journal - Multi-dimensional pain inventory - Pain information and beliefs questionnaire - Pain and impairment relationship scale - Pain cognition questionnaire - Pain beliefs and perceptions inventory - Coping strategies questionnaire - Pain disability index - Hospital anxiety and depression questionnaire (HAD scale)

Cognitive impairment

The presence of cognitive impairment makes pain assessment more difficult. The level of impairment is influential.

In people with difficulty in communication (including cognitive impairment) and in situations where procedures might cause pain, an observational assessment is additionally required. Health care professionals should familiarise themselves with the range of behaviours which may indicate the presence of pain. These behaviours differ between individuals and between pains: none are specific indicators of pain. Regular care-givers may be more sensitive to the meaning of behaviours, but it is important not to dismiss the possibility of pain without further attempts to assess it.

Evidence activity

 3.3 Commonly used methods of assessment and reasons for their use

What are the most commonly used methods of assessment and why are they used more?

3.4 Explain how to maintain regular pain relief

Actions that healthcare staff should take to maintain regular pain relief when supporting and caring for individuals in particular circumstances are set out below.

- **Responding to increased sleeping** – it is important that healthcare staff allow the individual to rest and sleep as required. However, when providing care for the individual healthcare staff should continue to talk to the individual and explain what they are going to do.

- **Skin care** – it is vital that healthcare staff continue to maintain the individual's personal hygiene according to the individual care plan. Discreetly check for incontinence. Ensuring that the skin remains clean, dry and free from pressure sores will reduce the risk of infection and promote comfort.

- **Pain relief** – healthcare staff can monitor the effectiveness of analgesia, requesting a review of medication when the individual appears to be experiencing breakthrough pain. When the individual is unable to swallow medication, rather than regularly administer injections a syringe driver may be used. This will administer the medication regularly over a 24-hour period without the need to regularly inject the individual, which may cause distress and discomfort. You should also observe the individual for unwanted side-effects of medication.

- **Supporting a person who is confused or disorientated** – healthcare staff can support the confused and disorientated individual by remaining calm, re-orientating them to time, place and person. It is important that staff do this sensitively. Giving too much information using words the individual does not understand can add to the confusion. Therefore, healthcare staff should use words/phrases the individual understands, give short concise explanations, and be prepared to frequently repeat information.

- **Food and fluid intake** – individuals should not be forced or pressured into eating or drinking. Healthcare staff should ensure that meals offered are appropriate to the individuals beliefs, e.g. do not offer meat to a vegetarian.

- **Swallowing** – healthcare staff should observe the individual for any swallowing difficulties, as this may lead to choking or inhalation of food and fluids into the lungs. If the individual is alert when swallowing difficulties occur and they wish to continue eating and drinking, they will need to be assessed by a speech therapist.

- **Mouth care** – if the individual is unable to meet their own mouth care needs, then healthcare staff should provide mouth care according to the individual's needs. Teeth and dentures should be cleaned regularly. Ice lollies, ice cubes, water-soaked swabs or a water spray may be used to keep the mouth moist. Petroleum jelly may be used to prevent the lips from cracking.

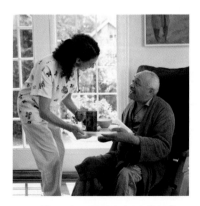

Figure 2.6 Food intake

The timing of pain relief

It is very important that pain relief is given at appropriate times. The type and dosage of pain medication will be determined by individual need. The ultimate goal should be that the person is comfortable and pain free at all times. Do not assume that all people will require the same amount and type of medication, even if they are at a similar stage of the same illness. Some people may only need medication occasionally. However, for the majority of people they will need regular medication to achieve relief of their pain. This medication could range from a mild analgesic such as paracetamol or a strong opiate such as diamorphine.

The purpose of giving medication on schedule is so the pain stays away. It becomes more difficult to treat pain once it returns. When pain relief is given regularly, oral medication can be as effective as that given by other routes (e.g. injection, trans-dermal-patches on the skin).

Pain medication, in palliative care, should be given at all times prescribed, every time, even if there is no pain.

Opiates should be prescribed regularly, either approximately four hourly or on a more long acting basis. e.g. 12/24 hourly. Opiates can be given orally unless the person suffers side effects, or has digestive tract problems or swallowing difficulties. Fentanyl patches last for three days, over which they continually release medication through the skin (trans-dermal). A syringe driver is a method by which a needle is placed under the skin and is attached to a syringe where a small battery operated pump delivers a continuous dosage of an opiate, such as diamorphine. The syringe is renewed usually every 24 hours. Other medication, such as an anti-emetic, can be given this way. The equipment is very small and can be carried in a holster or pouch, hidden under a person's clothing.

Pain relief should always be given prior to any activities that are known to, or it is anticipated that may cause, pain. Activities could be walking, certain treatments or therapies, renewing of dressings or positional changes. It is important to ensure analgesia has taken effect before the activity is attempted. If you are unsure always check with your manager.

The World Health Organisation has published a three step ladder to be used as general advice and guidance for care settings which adopt a step like approach to pain relief. This means that pain medication should be tailored to meet each individual's needs and should, generally, begin with a relatively low strength analgesic. This can be built up depending on the individual's needs.

Evidence activity

(3.4) Explain how to maintain regular pain relief

Explore the Analgesic Ladder and its effectiveness

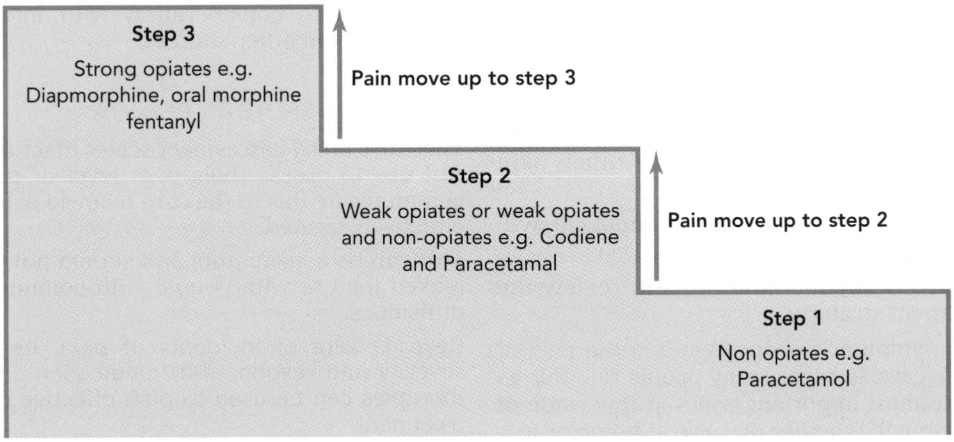

Step 3
Strong opiates e.g. Diapmorphine, oral morphine fentanyl

Pain move up to step 3

Step 2
Weak opiates or weak opiates and non-opiates e.g. Codiene and Paracetamal

Pain move up to step 2

Step 1
Non opiates e.g. Paracetamol

Figure 2.7 The Analgesic Ladder

LO4 Be able to integrate symptom management in the care management process

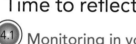 Explain how symptom management is an important part of the care planning process

When someone is dying, any type of pain can be significant and overwhelming; it may often be necessary to make a number of medication changes towards the end of an individual's life. A person's condition requires continual monitoring in order to enable a good level of pain/symptom control. Evaluating the effectiveness of medications forms an important part of individualised care at the end of life.

> ### Time to reflect
>
> **4.1** Monitoring in your setting
>
> How is monitoring carried out in your setting?

Pain is thought to be one of the commonest symptoms at the end of life, but dying people may suffer from many other symptoms. To allow accurate monitoring of changes, use a validated pain scale and use the same scale throughout. Always accept the patient's reported level of pain, even if it seems out of proportion.

This will allow appropriate selection of pain management strategies, according to the needs of the patient.

- Offer appropriate analgesic or other pain management.
- As the patient's condition changes so will their needs.
- If there is any increase in pain, review the treatment strategy.

Pain and symptom management is a big part of end of life care, because many people rate this as one of the most important issues at this stage of their treatment, whether they are at home or in a hospital or other assisted care. End of life care specialists liaise and work with all the parties involved to treat and manage pain and symptoms in a coordinated plan.

> ### Evidence activity
>
> **4.1** Using a pain scale
>
> Select a pain scale and use it. Does it meet assessment and monitoring needs?

4.2 Regularly monitor symptoms associated with end of life care

Observe the person and identify any changes in their verbal and non-verbal communication. Non-verbal signs are particularly important in people with communication difficulties such as, for example, speech, hearing, understanding or insight problems. This may mean they are unable to communicate their pain, discomfort and related stress by speech. Care workers must be aware that some people may not have the ability to communicate their pain or discomfort due to brain injury, disease or mental health problems. This is a particular problem in those people with dementia – who may become agitated, noisy and aggressive, as care professionals fail to recognise pain as the cause.

The use of gestures, facial expression and the written word can aid communication.

Discuss with individuals what their perception of the cause of their pain or discomfort is. For those people with communication difficulties, discussion may take place with family and friends, and others who know the individuals well. This, however, must not be the only assessment, but must be taken into consideration with information gathered from other sources.

Pain assessment scales

There are many assessment scales that the person can use to assess their own level of pain, and communicate this to the care team so pain can be effectively treated.

This can be a useful tool and should not be overlooked for use with people with communication difficulties.

Records kept of incidents of pain, its level of severity and responses to medication and other therapies can be used to plan effective care and treatment.

A tool that makes use of faces (Wong–Baker Tool) can be helpful in certain care settings; for example, settings for children or adults with some cognitive impairment or learning disability.

Keeping a pain diary can also be a good way of not only assessing pain, but also reviewing the effects of pain medication and other interventions.

The recording of all care and changes must adhere to the following basic principles:

- Handwriting must be legible and permanent.
- Dark ink should be used (so it will be clear when scanned or photocopied).
- All entries should be signed with a legible name and job title clearly stated.
- Entries should include the date and time.
- Records should be in chronological order, timely, concise and comprehensive.
- Do not leave 'white space' – draw a line through it to indicate that the entry is complete.
- Text should be clear, concise, unambiguous and accurate.

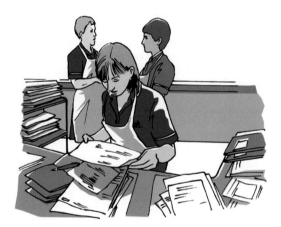

Figure 2.8 Monitoring records

Time to reflect

4.2 Review records you have completed

Review some records you have completed. Did you meet all of the identified requirements?

Evidence activity

4.2 Key records required for each person

What are the key records you are required to maintain for each person?

4.3 Report changes in symptoms according to policies in own work setting

The healthcare worker has a vital role to play in the management and control of distressing symptoms. Care workers should:

- Observe the person for any changes in condition or unusual signs or symptoms.
- Provide support.
- Give reassurance and whatever forms of therapy staff are trained to offer.
- Report and document findings.

Notes should be detailed and objective. Accurate descriptions strengthen documentation so use specific quantities, actual dates, time frames and distances and, where pertinent, use exact quotes from patients. Vague and meaningless expressions or clichés such as 'slept well', 'had a good day', 'up and about' should be avoided, as they do nothing to enhance communication between clinicians.

All entries must be factual and should not include jargon, abbreviations or irrelevant speculation. Many organisations have an approved list of abbreviations and only these should be used. Using unauthorised abbreviations can cause serious errors or, at the very least, waste people's time when trying to find out what they mean.

The individual's professional judgement must be used to decide what is relevant and should be recorded and what is unnecessary. Details of assessments and reviews should be recorded, with notes made of any risks identified or any problems that arose, with the actions taken to remedy the situation clearly stated. There is a duty to communicate fully with colleagues to ensure that they have all the information they need about patients.

How much is 'enough'? A general rule of thumb will be that any clinically significant information that shows the progression of the patient's care and condition must be evident in the documentation.

Unexpected events must be documented, together with what happened or was done as a follow-up to the event and commentary on the outcome. For example, when a patient complains of additional or worsening pain an entry should be made about what pain relief was provided, whether the pain subsided and whether the patient was satisfied with the intervention.

Records must not be destroyed or altered without authorisation and where alterations have been necessary they should be dated, timed and accompanied by the name, job title and signature of the person making the changes. Any alterations made must be clear and auditable and reflect the local organisation's policy. Under no circumstances should records be falsified.

Where possible, the patient and/or carer should be involved in the record-keeping process. It is important that the language used is understood by patients and colleagues and should not include coded expressions or sarcastic or humorous abbreviations to describe people being cared for. Value judgements, culturally insensitive comments and labelling that may imply discrimination must also be avoided.

The basic principles for record-keeping, accountability and safeguarding confidentiality apply to electronic records as well as paper-based systems. It is important to maintain the confidentiality of passwords and/or other access information by logging off when not using a system and taking necessary precautions to protect confidential information displayed on monitors.

Research and investigate

4.3 Legislation relating to the recording and storage of personal information

What legislation relates to the recording and storage of personal information?

Evidence activity

4.3 Using records in a court of law

When might records be used in a court of law? What needs to be considered if records are requested for this purpose?

4.4 Support the implementation of changes in the care plan

Care plans cover every aspect of a person's life. The purpose of a care plan is to provide a detailed written record of a client's needs and wishes and identify the level of support they require with their health, personal and social care needs in relation to end of life care.

Among other things, care plans cover:

- mobility
- continence
- washing and dressing
- social activities
- communication
- health.

In many organisations a care plan is updated daily by care or nursing staff.

In this case the care plan will include blank forms, which can be filled in to show the support the person has received that day and any changes in the client's condition. In other organisations daily information may be recorded in a separate book and then transferred to the care plan on a regular basis. In both cases the information that is recorded daily will be used to make appropriate changes to the care plan when it is reviewed. Therefore it is essential that the information you record is:

- legible, so that everyone can read what has been written
- accurate and factual
- complete, with all the necessary facts but without unnecessary waffle
- signed and dated, so that others can check with you if they have any questions about the information.

Being involved in the process of care planning helps people to maintain their independence and dignity. All individuals have a fundamental right to make decisions about their own lives, their needs and how they would like them to be met. The individual is central to the process of writing and monitoring care plans.

Receiving care can often make an older or disabled person feel that they are losing independence and can be damaging to a person's self-esteem. Involving people in care planning helps them to feel that they can still make decisions about their own lives. For adults with learning difficulties, promoting independence and improving everyday life skills is the ultimate goal of their care plan. One way of supporting this is to involve them in the decision-making process.

Evidence activity

 Implementing changes to care plans

Who else might be involved in implementing changes to a plan and why?

Assessment summary

Your reading of this chapter and completion of the activities will have prepared you to demonstrate your learning and understanding of end of life care. To achieve this unit, your assessor will require you to:

Learning outcomes	Assessment criteria
Learning outcome **1**: Understand the effects of symptoms in relation to end of life care by:	**1.1** identifying a range of conditions where you might provide end of life care See Evidence activity 1.1, p.30
	1.2 identifying common symptoms associated with end of life care See Evidence activity 1.2, p.31
	1.3 explaining how symptoms can cause an individual distress and discomfort See Evidence activity 1.3, p.32
	1.4 evaluating the significance of the individual's own perception of their symptoms See Evidence Activity 1.4, p.33
Learning outcome **2**: Be able to manage symptoms of end of life care by:	**2.1** demonstrating a range of techniques to provide symptom relief See Evidence activity 2.1, p.37
	2.2 describing own role in supporting therapeutic options used in symptom relief See Evidence activity 2.2, p.40
	2.3 responding to an individual's culture and beliefs in managing their symptoms See Evidence activity 2.3, p.41
	2.4 actively supporting the comfort and well-being in end of life care See Evidence activity 2.4, p.42
	2.5 recognising symptoms that identify the last few days of life may be approaching See Evidence activity 2.5, p.43

Learning outcomes	Assessment criteria
Learning outcome 3: Understand how to manage symptoms of pain by:	**3.1** identifying signs that may indicate that an individual is experiencing pain See Evidence activity 3.1, p.44
	3.2 describing factors that can influence an individual's perception of pain See Evidence activities 3.2, p.44
	3.3 describing a range of assessment tools for monitoring pain in individuals, including those with cognitive impairment See Evidence activity 3.3, p.46
	3.4 explaining how to maintain regular pain relief See Evidence activity 3.4, p.47
Learning outcome 4: Be able to integrate symptom management in the care management process by:	**4.1** explaining how symptom management is an important part of the care planning process See Evidence activity 4.1, p.48
	4.2 regularly monitoring symptoms associated with end of life care See Evidence activity 4.2, p.49
	4.3 reporting changes in symptoms according to policies and procedures in own work settings See Evidence activity 4.3, p.50
	4.4 supporting the implementation of changes in the care plan See Evidence activity 4.4, p.51

Good luck!

Web links

Alzheimer's Society	www.alzheimers.org.uk
Care Quality Commission (CQC)	www.cqc.org.uk
Cruse Bereavement Care	www.crusebereavementcare.org.uk
Department of Health	www.dh.gov.uk
Huntington's Disease Association	www.hda.org.uk
Macmillan Cancer Support	www.macmillan.org.uk
Marie Curie Cancer Care	www.mariecurie.org.uk
Multiple Sclerosis Society	www.mssociety.org.uk
National Council for Palliative Care	www.ncpc.org.uk
National End of Life Care Programme	www.endoflifecareforadults.nhs.uk
Parkinson's Disease Society	www.parkinsons.org.uk
The Motor Neurone Disease Association	www.mndassociation.org
Princess Royal Trust for Carers	www.carers.org

3

For Unit EOL 303
Understand advance care planning

What are you finding out?

An early assessment of an individual's needs and wishes as they approach the end of life is vital to establish their preferences and choices and identify any areas of unmet need. It is important to explore the physical, psychological, social, spiritual, cultural and, where appropriate, environmental needs / wishes of each individual.

People approaching the end of their life frequently have complex, wide-ranging and changing needs. Meeting these needs requires effective care coordination across boundaries, supported by strong communication between the different teams involved in providing care. First and foremost, it calls for a sound understanding of the individual's needs, preferences and priorities for care.

The reading and activities in this chapter will help you to:

- Understand the principles of advance care planning

- Understand the person centred approach to advance care planning

- Understand when advance care planning may be required

LO1 Understand the principles of advance care planning

1.1 Describe the difference between a care or support plan and an Advance Care Plan

Advance care planning (ACP) is a process of discussion between an individual and their care providers irrespective of discipline.

The difference between ACP and planning more generally is that the process of ACP is to make clear a person's wishes and will usually take place in the context of an anticipated deterioration in the individual's condition in the future, with attendant loss of capacity to make decisions and/or ability to communicate wishes to others. This may lead to making an advance statement, an Advance Decision to Refuse Treatment (ADRT), a Do Not Attempt Cardiopulmonary Resuscitation (DNACPR) decision, or other types of decision (such as making a Lasting Power of Attorney).

Advance care planning is a process enabling a patient to express wishes about their future healthcare in consultation with their healthcare providers, family members and other important people in their lives. Based on the ethical principle of patient autonomy and the legal doctrine of patient consent, advance care planning helps to ensure that the concept of consent is respected if the patient becomes incapable of participating in treatment decisions.

Evidence activity

1.1 Differences between a care or support plan and an advance care plan

List the key differences between a care or support plan and an advance care plan

1.2 Explain the purpose of advance care planning

According to the Department of Health, 'End of life care is care that helps all those with advanced, progressive, incurable illness to live as well as possible until they die. It enables the supportive and palliative care needs of both patient and family to be identified and met throughout the last phase of life and into bereavement. It includes management of pain and other symptoms and provision of psychological, social, spiritual and practical support.'

The **holistic** common assessment process offers an opportunity to explore the individual's wider needs and identify what action should be taken to meet them. There should be a strong focus throughout on supporting choice and decision making and on helping people to identify and achieve the outcomes they want for themselves, wherever possible.

Key terms

Holistic refers to the treatment of the whole person, taking into account mental and social factors, rather than just the physical.

It is vital to make an early assessment of an individual's needs and wishes as they approach the end of life to establish their preferences and choices and identify any areas of unmet need. The physical, psychological, social, spiritual, cultural and, where appropriate, environmental needs/wishes of each individual should be explored. People who are approaching the end of their life often have complex, wide-ranging and changing needs. Meeting those needs requires effective care coordination across boundaries, supported by strong communication between the different teams involved in providing care. It calls for a sound understanding of the individual's needs, preferences and priorities for care. Effective holistic assessment processes are key to this: the need for these was identified in NICE's 'Guidance on Cancer Services: Improving Supportive and Palliative Care for Adults with Cancer', published in 2004. Since then, the national 'End of Life Care Strategy' (for England) highlighted the importance of ensuring all adults requiring end of life care receive holistic assessment – encompassing physical, psychological, social, cultural, environmental, spiritual and financial needs – to support delivery of high quality care during this last phase of life.

Nevertheless, challenges persist in delivering holistic assessment. Some individuals' needs are never adequately assessed; some assessment is only partial, restricted to physical needs alone, for example. Other individuals undergo repeated assessments of the same aspects by different professionals in different settings, with information rarely shared between the teams. This can be tiring and frustrating for individuals and their families, at a point when energy is limited and time is precious; it is also a poor use of NHS and social care resources.

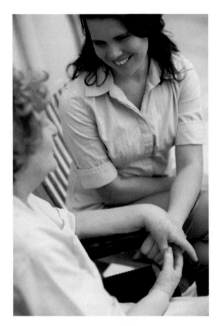

Figure 3.1 Meeting holistic needs

It is now recognised that a person has needs beyond their physical care; therefore, it is important that the whole care needs of the person are met. Care should be planned to take into consideration the religious, spiritual, psychological, social and cultural as well as physical needs. This means looking at individuals as a whole person rather than just focusing on their medical condition.

Many people, both within and outside your care organisation, will contribute to the care of the dying in a variety of ways. The most obvious responsibility of the team in which you work is the responsibility to deliver the highest standard of holistic care to the individual, with each team member providing their own aspect of care.

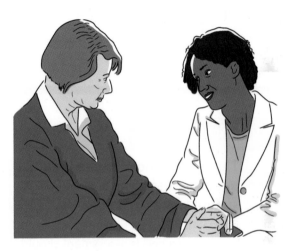

Figure 3.2 Spiritual needs

Time to reflect

1.2 **Your needs and your personal experiences of receiving medical advice or treatment**

Think about a time when you, or someone you know, received medical advice or treatment. Were all their needs considered or just the particular issue at the time?

Within your setting there should be members of staff with experience and training in looking after people who are dying, who can advise other members of staff in the support of these individuals. In nursing homes, there should be nursing staff with appropriate skills in end of life care. All care staff should receive some training in looking after people who are dying and be aware of their physical, spiritual and emotional needs, in order to facilitate a holistic approach to care. It is vital that care staff should also only act within their level of competence, and should know when and how to call upon other members of the team for support.

A combined approach to holistic common assessment helps by creating opportunities for the individual to consider, alongside those involved in their care, all aspects affecting their life, and to identify and articulate their needs and priorities. It helps to put that individual in control, while prompting other agencies to take action when required. Through effective record storing and sharing, it minimises duplication, helps avoid unnecessary repeated assessments, and contributes to effective care planning. Above all, it should result in a better experience of end of life care for the individual, promoting dignity and choice in the final phase of life.

An assessment may be carried out in any physical setting that ensures comfort and privacy. The place of assessment will be determined by the person's care setting at that key point in their pathway.

Person-centred care aims to treat the individual holistically, recognising that all individuals have a right to respect; being treated with dignity and consideration of their wishes, regardless of their illness. Usually the term person-centred care is linked with the care of people with dementia. However, its principles can be applied to anyone with a life-limiting illness.

Historically, a person's illness or condition was at the centre of care, upon which treatment and care plans were based. End of life care adopts the principles of a person-centred approach, thus placing the needs and feelings of the person at the centre, around which everything else is based.

Research and investigate

 1.2 Find out about what is involved in the person-centred approach and explain how this differs from previous approaches

What is involved in the person-centred approach and how does this differ from previous approaches?

Evidence activity

1.2 Think about how to carry out a needs assessment and create a suitable form to use in an assessment

Think about how a needs assessment should be carried out. What do you need to include? Who do you need to consult and how would you go about this? Prepare a form you could use, considering all aspects discussed.

1.3 Identify the national, local and organisational agreed ways of working for advance care planning

Advance care planning (ACP) is a voluntary process of discussion and review to help an individual who has capacity to anticipate how their condition may affect them in the future and, if they wish, set on record choices about their care and treatment and/or an advance decision to refuse a treatment in specific circumstances, so that these can be referred to by those responsible for their care or treatment (whether professional staff or family carers) in the event that they lose capacity to decide once their illness progresses. The legal context of advance care planning varies across the world. In the United Kingdom, under the terms of the Mental Capacity Act 2005, formalised outcomes of advance care planning might include one or more of the following:

i. advance statements to inform subsequent best-interests decisions

ii. advance decisions to refuse treatment which are legally binding if valid and applicable to the circumstances at hand

iii. appointment of Lasting Powers of Attorney ('health and welfare' and/or 'property and affairs').

Not everyone will wish to make such records. Less formally, the person may wish to name someone whom they wish to be consulted if they lose capacity. These are only relevant to the care and treatment to a person once they have lost capacity to make decision(s) about the issues they cover.

The key principles of the advance care planning process are as follows:

- The process is voluntary. No pressure should be brought to bear by the professional, the family or any organisation on the individual concerned to take part in ACP.

- ACP must be a patient-centred dialogue over a period of time.

- The process of ACP is a reflection of society's desire to respect personal autonomy.

- The content of any discussion should be determined by the individual concerned.

- The individual may not wish to confront future issues; this should be respected.

- All health and social care staff should be open to any discussion, which may be instigated by an individual, and know how to respond to their questions.

- Health and social care staff should instigate ACP only if, in the context of a professional judgement, that leads them to believe it is likely to benefit the care of the individual. The discussion should be introduced sensitively.

- Staff will require the appropriate training to enable them to communicate effectively and to understand the legal and ethical issues involved.

- Staff need to be aware when they have reached the limits of their knowledge and competence, and know when and from whom to seek advice.

- Discussion should focus on the views of the individual, although they may wish to invite their carer or another close family member or friend to participate. Some families may have discussed their issues and would welcome an approach to share this discussion.

- Confidentiality should be respected in line with current good practice and professional guidance.
- Health and social care staff should be aware of and give a realistic account of the support, services and choices available in the particular circumstances. This should entail referral to an appropriate colleague or agency when necessary.
- The professional must have adequate knowledge of the benefits, harms and risk.
- Choice in terms of place of care will influence treatment options, as certain treatments may not be available at home or in a care home, e.g. chemotherapy or intravenous therapy. Individuals may need to be admitted to hospital for symptom management, or may need to be admitted to a hospice or hospital, because support is not available at home
- ACP requires that the individual has the capacity to understand, discuss options available and agree to what is then planned. Agreement should be documented.
- Should an individual wish to make a decision to refuse treatment (advance decision) they should be guided by a professional with appropriate knowledge and this should be documented according to the requirements of the MCA 2005. www.legislation.gov.uk/ukpga/2005/9/contents

 Explain the legal position of an advance care plan

For individuals with capacity, it is their current wishes about their care which need to be considered. Under the Mental Capacity Act (MCA) 2005, individuals can continue to anticipate future decision making about their care or treatment should they lack capacity. In this context, the outcome may be the completion of a statement of wishes and preferences or, if referring to refusal of specific treatment, may lead onto an advance decision to refuse treatment (Chapter 9 MCA 2005 Code of Practice). This is not mandatory or automatic and will depend on the person's wishes. Alternatively, an individual may decide to appoint a person to represent them by choosing a person (an 'attorney') to take decisions on their behalf if they subsequently lose capacity (Chapter 5 MCA 2005 Code of Practice).

Time to reflect

1.4 Mental Capacity Act 2005

Try to think of a time when the Mental Capacity Act 2005 may be used.

Time to reflect

1.3 Your priorities when reviewing needs and planning for the future

What would be your priority when reviewing needs and planning for the future?

A statement of wishes and preferences is not legally binding. However, it does have legal standing and must be taken into account when making a judgement in a person's best interests. Careful account needs to be taken of the relevance of statements of wishes and preferences when making best-interest decisions (Chapter 5 MCA 2005 Code of Practice). If an advance decision to refuse treatment has been made, it is a legally binding document if that advance decision can be shown to be valid and applicable to the current circumstances. If it relates to life-sustaining treatment it must be a written document, which is signed and witnessed.

Evidence activity

 Explain who should be involved in recording advance care plans and why

Who should be involved in recording advance care plans and why?

Evidence activity

 Explain what rights a person has under the MCA

Carry out research into the MCA 2005 Code of Practice. What rights does a person have under the MCA?

1.5 Explain what is involved in an 'Advance Decision to Refuse Treatment'

It is a general principle of law and medical practice that people have a right to consent to, or refuse, treatment. The courts have recognised that adults have the right to say in advance that they want to refuse treatment if they lose capacity in the future – even if this results in their death. A valid and applicable advance decision to refuse treatment has the same force as a contemporaneous decision. This has been a fundamental principle of the common law for many years and it is now set out in the Act. Sections 24–26 of the Mental Capacity Act set out when a person can make an advance decision to refuse treatment.

This applies if:

- the person is 18 or older, and
- they have the capacity to make an advance decision about treatment.

Healthcare professionals must follow an advance decision if it is valid and applies to the particular circumstances. If they do not, they could face criminal prosecution (they could be charged for committing a crime) or civil liability (somebody could sue them). Advance decisions can have serious consequences for the people who make them. They can also have an important impact on family and friends, and professionals involved in their care. Before healthcare professionals can apply an advance decision, there must be proof that the decision exists, is valid and is applicable to the current circumstances.

People can only make advance decisions to refuse treatment. Nobody has the right to demand specific treatment, either at the time or in advance. So, no one can insist on being given treatments that healthcare professionals consider to be clinically unnecessary, futile or inappropriate. However, people can make a request or state their wishes and preferences in advance. Healthcare professionals should then consider the request when deciding what is in the patient's best interests if the patient lacks capacity.

For most people, there will be no doubt about their capacity to make an advance decision. Even those who lack capacity to make some decisions may have the capacity to make an advance decision. In some cases, it may be helpful to have evidence of a person's capacity to make the advance decision (e.g. if there is a risk that it may be challenged in the future). It is also important to remember that capacity can change over time and a person who lacks capacity to make a decision now might be able to make it in the future.

Time to reflect

1.5 Persuading people to be more open about discussing death and dying

Do you and your family and friends have difficulties discussing death and dying? How can we persuade people to be a little more open about this?

There are no particular requirements about the format of an advance decision. It can be written or verbal unless it deals with life-sustaining treatment, in which case it must be written and specific rules apply.

An advance decision to refuse treatment:

- must state precisely what treatment is to be refused – a statement giving a general desire not to be treated is not enough
- may set out the circumstances when the refusal should apply
- will only apply at a time when the person lacks capacity to consent to, or refuse, specific treatment.

People can use medical language or everyday language in their advance decision. However, they must make clear what their wishes are and what treatment they would like to refuse.

There is not a set form for written advance decisions. Content will vary depending on a person's wishes and situation. However, it should include the following information:

- full details of the person making the advance decision, including date of birth and home address
- the name and address of the person's GP and whether they have a copy of the document
- a statement that the document should be used if the person ever lacks capacity to make treatment decisions
- a clear statement of the decision, the treatment to be refused and the circumstances in which the decision will apply
- the date the document was written (or reviewed)
- the person's signature (or the signature of someone that the person has asked to sign on their behalf and in their presence)
- the signature of the person witnessing the signature, if there is one (or a statement directing somebody to sign on the person's behalf).

Evidence activity

1.5 **Key points relating to advance decisions contained in the 'End of Life Care Strategy', 2008**

Research the Department of Health's 'End of Life Care Strategy', 2008 and highlight key points relating to advance decisions.

1.6 **Explain what is meant by a 'Do Not Attempt Cardiopulmonary Resuscitation' order (DNACPR)**

A Do Not Attempt Cardiopulmonary Resuscitation order (DNACPR) is a legal order which tells a medical team not to perform cardio pulmonary resuscitation (CPR) on a patient. However, this does not affect other medical treatments.

Decisions relating to a DNACPR must be made on the basis of an individual assessment of each case. Advance care planning for DNACPR decisions is an important part of good clinical care for those at risk of cardiac arrest. It is not necessary to initiate discussions about DNACPR decisions if there is no reason to believe that the person may suffer a cardiac arrest, and CPR must be attempted if no DNACPR decision has been made and formally recorded.

If CPR would not restart the heart and breathing it should not be attempted.

Where the benefits of CPR may be outweighed by the burdens, the person's informed views are of paramount importance. If the person lacks capacity, those close to the patient should be involved in discussions to explore the patient's wishes, feelings, beliefs and values.

If a patient with capacity refuses CPR, or a patient lacking capacity has a valid and applicable advance decision refusing CPR, this should be respected.

Decision-making capacity refers to the ability that individuals possess to make decisions or to take actions that influence their life. In a legal context it refers to a person's ability to do something, including making a decision which may have legal consequences for the person or for other people. Patients over 16 years of age are presumed to have capacity to make their own decisions unless there is evidence to the contrary.

■ **Research and investigate**

1.6 **Find out about CPR**

Find out how CPR is carried out.

CPR must not be attempted if it is contrary to valid and applicable advance decisions made when the patient has capacity. Advance decisions are covered by the Mental Capacity Act 2005 (in England and Wales). The Act confirms that an advance decision refusing CPR will be valid and, therefore, legally binding on the healthcare team if:

• The patient was 18 years or over and had capacity when the decision was made.

• The decision is in writing, signed and witnessed.

• It includes a statement that the decision is to apply even if the patient's life is at risk.

• The advance decision has not been withdrawn.

• The patient has not, since the advance decision was made, appointed a welfare attorney to make decisions about CPR on their behalf.

• The patient has not done anything that is clearly inconsistent with its terms.

• The circumstances that have arisen match those envisaged in the advance decision.

If an advance decision does not meet the criteria, but appears to set out a clear indication of the patient's wishes, it will not be legally binding, but should be taken into consideration in determining the patient's best wishes. Although advance decisions often do not come to light until an individual has lost capacity, there should be a presumption that the individual had capacity when an advance decision was made, unless there are grounds to suspect otherwise.

The decision

There is no legal or ethical requirement to discuss resuscitation status with all the patients, or with those close to patients who lack capacity, if the risk of cardiac arrest is considered low as this could cause undue stress and anxiety.

In some cases, the DNACPR decision is a straightforward clinical one. If the clinical team believe that CPR will not restart the heart and maintain breathing, it should not be offered or attempted.

CPR (which can cause harm in some situations) should not be attempted if it will not be successful. However the patient's individual circumstances and the most up-to-date guidance must be considered carefully before such a decision is made.

One individual needs to take charge of ensuring that the decision is made properly, is recorded and is conveyed to all those who need to know it.

The overall responsibility for the DNACPR decision rests with the consultant in charge of the patient's care. However, it is good practice to seek the views of other members of the health-care team. These team members could be from primary or secondary care settings and be from a medical or nursing background.

With due regard to the patient's expressed wishes and confidentiality, the view of people close to the patient should also be sought.

Teamwork and good communication are of paramount importance; taking confidentiality into account the consultant psychiatrist should always be prepared to discuss a DNACPR decision with any other health professional, relative or carer involved in the patient's care.

Recording decisions

The health and social care records must show clear documentation of decisions. These records must include:

- the decision
- information on how the decision was made and who was involved
- the date of the decision
- the reason for the decision
- the name and position of person responsible for making the decision.

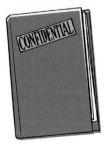

Figure 3.3 Confidentiality

Review

DNACPR decisions must be reviewed:

- at least weekly
- whenever a change occurs in the patient's condition
- if the patient requests it.

These reviews must be clearly documented in the contemporaneous health and social care records, with the rationale for continuation/change being recorded and the names of those involved in the discussions highlighted.

> ### Evidence activity
>
>
>
> **(1.6) Create a form which could be used to record information relating to a DNACPR decision**
>
> Create a form which could be used to record information relating to a DNACPR decision. What should the form contain and why?

LO2 Understand the process of advance care planning

(2.1) Explain when advance care planning may be introduced

Advance care planning is a voluntary process of discussion and review to help an individual who has capacity to anticipate how their condition may affect them in the future and, if they wish, set on record choices about their care and treatment and/or an advance decision to refuse a treatment in specific circumstances, so that these can be referred to by those responsible for their care or treatment (whether professional staff or family carers) in the event that they lose capacity to decide once their illness progresses.

Advance care planning describes the process of discussion between individuals and their care providers about the individual's preferences and priorities for their future care. Advance care planning is particularly important for people with a life-limiting condition, as they are likely to deteriorate in the future and may then lack capacity or be unable to communicate their wishes to others. Advance care planning discussions may include exploration of the type of care that individuals would wish to receive in the future, their preferred place of care and their views on future hospital admission. More specific topics which may be explored by healthcare professionals include the person's understanding of their illness, their prognosis and the benefits or appropriateness of intensive or emergency treatments. Any discussion should be introduced sensitively by professionals with the necessary communication skills. The person may choose to involve carers, friends and family in the discussion(s). It is important to note that not everyone will want to have these discussions and they should not be forced to do so.

Research and investigate

2.1 Find out about the key priorities for discussion in advance care planning

Try to find out what key priorities might be discussed when advance care planning.

Advance care planning is a process of discussion between an individual and their care provider, irrespective of discipline. The difference between advance care planning and more general planning is that the aim of the process of advance care planning is to make clear a person's wishes and will usually take place in the context of an anticipated deterioration of the individual's condition. It is recommended that with the individual's agreement this discussion is documented, regularly reviewed and communicated to key persons involved in their care. Advance care planning may be instigated by either the individual, or a care provider at any time, not necessarily in the context of illness progression but may be at one of the following key points in the individual's life:

* when a patient chooses
* when diagnosed as palliative, possibly in a clinic environment
* before admission to care home
* before admission to hospital or hospice
* if acute episode occurs (e.g. diagnosis of extensive malignant spinal cord compression)
* if there is other significant emotional, physical, social, psychological or spiritual change in patient circumstances.

The national guides indicate that any discipline may be involved in the process of discussion and documentation; however, for specific medical or social decisions, discussion with senior medical, nursing and social care staff may be more appropriate (e.g. for an Advance Decision to Refuse Treatment – ADRT). Patients may need to be asked if they have a completed Statement of Preference and Wishes, an ADRT or LPA (personal welfare).

It is essential to consider the ongoing process of advance care planning as the patient moves between health and social care providers.

There needs to be clarity that advance care planning is about the patient's wishes. Patients should be encouraged to include relatives in their discussions and decisions, remembering that relatives can only make choices on behalf of the patient if they hold a valid and registered Lasting Power of Attorney for Personal Welfare (i.e. if permission has been given for them to refuse or consent to life-sustaining treatments). It is good practice to involve families and carers in making decisions when a patient has lost capacity, asking them to consider what they think their relative might have wanted (not what they want for their relative) if it has not been documented.

Evidence activity

2.1 Providing a summary of the advance care plan for carers, relatives and friends of the person involved

Provide a brief summary of the advance care plan which can be easily understood by carers, relatives and friends of the person involved.

 2.2 ## Outline who might be involved in the advance care planning process

Advance care planning is a voluntary process of discussion about future care between an individual and their care providers, irrespective of discipline. If the individual wishes, their family and friends may be included. It is recommended that with the individual's agreement this discussion is documented, regularly reviewed, and communicated to key persons involved in their care. The term connects with 'care planning', a stage in the process of care management which involves discussing with service users and carers the various options and putting them together in an agreed written plan. In end of life care planning is often seen, particularly by doctors and nurses, as limited to the process of creating 'advance directives'; that is, legally enforceable statements of the patient's wishes not to receive particular treatments. Patients cannot of course say in advance in a legally enforceable way that they want a particular treatment; deciding on appropriate treatment in the best interests of their patient is the doctor's role.

The difference between advance care planning and care planning is that the process of ACP can only involve someone with capacity to decide and usually takes place in the context of an anticipated deterioration in the individual's condition in the future, with attendant loss of capacity to make decisions and/or the ability to communicate wishes to others. Although advance care planning is often focused on informing decisions once a person has lost capacity, the process can help a person with life-limiting illness to consider clinical or personal arrangements for the future progression of their illness which are not specific to anticipation of loss of capacity. To this extent, advance care planning is part of the wider care planning process.

People may need support to make advance care plans. This support could come from family, friends, care staff or doctors. You should not assume that people already know about advance care plans – many people are not aware of them. Remember too that advance care planning discussions with a person with dementia will take time. It is unlikely that a one-off conversation or meeting will cover everything.

Evidence activity

 2.2 Who might be involved in advance care planning

List the professionals you think might be involved in an advance care plan.

 2.3 Describe the type of information an individual may need to enable them to make informed decisions

It is very important that people who are nearing the end of their life feel respected and valued. Health and social care staff have a major role in ensuring this happens. First and foremost, it is essential to realise that the person is a multifaceted being with unique experiences, qualities, values and needs.

It is essential to remember that a person who is nearing the end of their life has the same basic human rights as other people, and this should always be respected. In addition, throughout the end of life care period, these people also have a right to:

- a high standard of care
- make choices
- be given explanations in order that they can make informed choices
- be treated with dignity and afforded their privacy
- have their cultural and religious beliefs respected
- have their physical and psychological needs addressed in the course of their daily care
- be as independent as possible
- be safe and secure
- freedom of movement.

Considering the rights of individuals is one of the core concepts of delivering care that is person centred

Partnership working is an essential aspect in supporting people who are nearing the end of their life. The partners that you work with may include:

- the individuals you support, their carers, family and friends
- your colleagues and other members of the immediate care team
- members of the specialist palliative care team
- hospital staff
- the individual's GP
- advocacy services.

The most important people in partnership working are the individuals you support and the people who are important to them. If these people feel they are actively participating in the partnership, this can have a dramatic effect on their overall health and well being. Partnership working with these key people will also help you to view and understand things from the perspective of the service user, which in essence leads to the delivery of care that is person centred.

Research and investigate

2.3 Find out about the various types of advocates, how to access them and their limitations

What types of advocates are there? How can they be accessed and what are the limitations of their role?

The use of advocates

The word advocacy is derived from the latin 'advocare', which means 'to call to one's aid'. It is concerned with standing up for an individual or group who are unable to do this themselves. An advocate therefore helps service users to express their needs and wishes.

If a person needs support with making choices about their care or expressing their views, they should be able to use a free advocacy service. Advocates:

• are independent of health and social care services

• support the person with decision making and speaking for themselves

• represent the views of people who are unable to represent their own views.

Good independent advocacy services can play an important part in people's self-directed support. And by helping individuals to express their views and get problems addressed, they can lead to changes that benefit others in similar situations.

The Mental Capacity Act also set up the Independent Mental Capacity Advocate (IMCA) service. This service helps vulnerable people who cannot make some (or all) important decisions about their lives. The IMCA service means that certain people who lack capacity will be helped to make difficult decisions; for example, in relation to medical treatment choices or where they live and choose to die. It is aimed at people who do not have relatives or friends to speak for them. A lack of mental capacity could be due to:

• a stroke or brain injury

• a mental health problem

• a dementia-related condition

• a learning disability

• unconsciousness.

 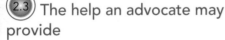

Time to reflect

2.3 The help an advocate may provide

How helpful do you think an advocate would be to a person?

Advocacy services are crucial when people are more vulnerable because, for example, they have learning difficulties or are being treated under a section of the Mental Health Act. Advocacy services may need to be called upon when a person has been assessed as lacking capacity. Health and social care workers must always assume a person has capacity to make decisions unless an assessment has proven that the ability to make decisions is lacking.

A person's capacity may need to be assessed if there is a particular situation where a decision needs to be made. The assessment would usually be undertaken by a care professional such as a doctor, a nurse or social worker where decisions about treatment, care or accommodation need to be made.

According to the Mental Capacity Act, in order to assess capacity, there are two questions that need to be answered.

• Question 1: Is there an impairment of or disturbance in the functioning of a person's mind or brain? If so:

• Question 2: Is the impairment or disturbance sufficient that the person lacks the capacity to make a particular decision?

A person is assessed as lacking the ability to make a decision if they cannot do one or more of the following:

• understand information presented to them about the decision

• retain the information for long enough to make the decision

• use or weigh up the information as part of the decision-making process

• communicate their decision by any means, for example, by talking, using sign language, squeezing a hand or blinking.

Before deciding that the person lacks capacity, the assessor must have tried to find ways of communicating with the person. Discussion should also take place with the person's family, friends, carers and other people in their support network.

An individual may be assigned an Independent Mental Capacity Advocate if the person is over the age of 16 years, has no support or representation and lacks capacity to make decisions in relation to medical treatment, a long-term care move, adult protection procedures or a care review.

Evidence activity

2.3 A case study approach to identifying a person who cannot participate in decision making and explaining how their needs can be best supported

Develop a case study identifying a person who cannot participate in decision making. How can their needs be best supported?

2.4 Explain how to use legislation to support decision-making about the capacity of an individual to take part in advance care planning

Capacity refers to the ability to make a decision about a particular issue at the time the decision needs to be made, or to give consent to a particular act. Assessing capacity and maximising capacity are essential aspects of the care planning process. It is important to appreciate that only people who have capacity can participate in advance care planning.

Advance care planning embraces the care of people with and without capacity to make their own decisions. It involves a process of assessment and person-centred dialogue to establish the person's needs, preferences and goals of care, and making decisions about how to meet these in the context of available resources. It can be oriented towards meeting immediate needs, as well as predicting future needs and making appropriate arrangements or contingency plans to address these.

Where a person lacks capacity to decide, care planning must focus on determining their best interests (through consultation with the person's companions and key professional carers) and making decisions to protect these. Any information about what the person's views might have been should be taken into account when trying to work out what is in their best interests. If any advance statements exist, which the person made before losing capacity, these should be taken into account in the process of determining best interests. If a person who has lost capacity has a valid and applicable advance decision to refuse treatment (ADRT) and/or has registered Lasting Powers of Attorney (LPA), these must be respected. Anything done under the authority of the LPA must be in the person's best interests.

If a person who lacks capacity has no close family or friends and has not recorded any choices about their care and treatment or made an advance decision to refuse treatment in advance of losing capacity, then an Independent Mental Capacity Advocate (IMCA) should be instructed and consulted regarding decision making about serious medical treatment, or about placement in hospital for longer than 28 days, or a care home for longer than 8 weeks. IMCAs may also have a role in case reviews or adult protection cases, where no one else is available to be consulted.

Advance care planning is the process of discussion between an individual and their care providers in order to make clear a person's wishes in the anticipation of deterioration in the future and attendant loss of capacity to make decisions or communicate. Advance care planning may include a Statement of Preferences and Wishes (e.g. preferred priorities of care) and/or an Advance Decision to Refuse Treatment (ADRT). Consideration may also need to be given to Lasting Power of Attorney (Personal Welfare) and the Best Interests principles.

Advance care planning centres on discussions with a person who has capacity to make decisions about their care and treatment. If the individual wishes, their family and friends may be included. It is recommended that with the individual's agreement discussions are documented, regularly reviewed, and communicated to key persons involved in their care.

Under the terms of the Mental Capacity Act 2005, formalised outcomes of advance care planning might include one or more of the following:

i) advance statements to inform subsequent best interests decisions;

ii) advance decisions to refuse treatment which are legally binding if valid and applicable to the circumstances at hand;

iii) appointment of Lasting Powers of Attorney ('health and welfare' and/or 'property and affairs').

Two key statutory principles of the Mental Capacity Act 2005 are:

- A person must be assumed to have capacity unless it is established that they lack capacity;

- A person is not to be treated as unable to make a decision unless all practicable steps to help them to do so have been taken without success.

Time to reflect

2.4 Involving others in your decision making

Think about a time when you had to make decisions. Who else did you involve? How did you feel about involving others?

Evidence activity

2.5 Communication in advance care planning

Reflect on a time when you perhaps did not have enough time or the ability to communicate what you wanted. How did this make you feel? What did you do?

Evidence activity

2.4 Needs assessment

Think about how a needs assessment should be carried out. What do you need to include? Who do you need to consult and how would you go about this? Prepare a form you could use; considering all aspects discussed.

2.6

Explain the meaning of informed consent

Consent is the principle that a person must give their permission before they receive any type of medical treatment. Consent is required from a patient regardless of the type of treatment being undertaken, from a blood test to an organ donation.

The principle of consent is one of the cornerstones of medical ethics. It is also enshrined (held sacred) in international human rights law. Informed consent is a legal procedure to ensure that a person knows all of the risks and costs involved in a treatment. The elements of informed consent include informing the client of the nature of the treatment, possible alternative treatments, and the potential risks and benefits of the treatment. In order for informed consent to be considered valid, the person must be competent and the consent should be given voluntarily.

What constitutes consent?

For consent to be valid, it must be voluntary and informed, and the person consenting must have the capacity to make the decision. These terms are explained below.

- **Voluntary**: the decision to consent or not consent to treatment must be made alone, and must not be due to pressure by medical staff, friends or family.

- **Informed**: the person must be given full information about what the treatment involves, including the benefits and risks, whether there are reasonable alternative treatments, and what will happen if treatment does not go ahead.

- **Capacity**: the person must be capable of giving consent, which means that they understand the information given to them, and they can use it to make an informed decision.

2.5

Explain how the individual's capacity to discuss advance care planning may influence their role in the process

The difference between advance care planning and care planning is that the process of ACP can only involve someone with capacity to decide and usually takes place in the context of an anticipated deterioration in the individual's condition in the future, with attendant loss of capacity to make decisions and/or the ability to communicate wishes to others. Although advance care planning is often focused on informing decisions once a person has lost capacity, the process can help a person with life-limiting illness to consider clinical or personal arrangements for the future progression of their illness which are not specific to anticipation of loss of capacity. To this extent, advance care planning is part of the wider care planning process.

People may need support to make advance care plans. This support could come from family, friends, care staff or doctors. You should not assume that people already know about advance care plans – many people are not aware of them. Remember too that advance care planning discussions with a person with dementia will take time. It is unlikely that a one-off conversation or meeting will cover everything.

There are a few exceptions when treatment can go ahead without consent and one main exception is if a person does not have the mental capacity (the ability to understand and use information) to make a decision about their treatment. In this case, the healthcare professionals can go ahead and give treatment if they believe that it is in the person's best interests.

The Mental Health Act (1983) sets out various legal rights that apply to people with severe mental health problems. The Act also contains the powers which, in extreme cases, enable some people with mental health problems to be compulsorily detained in hospital. The Mental Capacity Act (2005) is designed to protect people who cannot make decisions for themselves. The Act explains when a person is considered to be lacking capacity, and how decisions should be made in their best interests.

The Court of Protection is the legal body that oversees the operation of the Mental Capacity Act (2005).

An advance decision (previously called an advance directive) is a legally binding document that sets out in advance the treatments and procedures that someone does or does not consent to.

Having the capacity to consent

Under the terms of the Mental Capacity Act (2005), all adults are presumed to have sufficient capacity (the ability to use and understand information to make a decision) to decide on their own medical treatment unless there is significant evidence to suggest otherwise.

The evidence has to show that:

- a person's mind or brain is impaired or disturbed, and
- the impairment or disturbance means that the person is unable to make a decision at the current time.

Examples of impairments or disturbances in the mind or brain include:

- mental health conditions, such as schizophrenia (a condition that causes hallucinations and delusions) or bipolar disorder (manic depression – when an individual's moods swing from one extreme to another)
- dementia (an ongoing decline of mental abilities, such as memory and understanding)
- serious learning disabilities
- long-term effects of brain damage

- physical or mental conditions that cause confusion, drowsiness or a loss of consciousness
- delirium (mental confusion)
- intoxication caused by drug or alcohol misuse.

Someone is thought to be unable to make a decision if they are unable to:

- understand information about the decision
- remember that information
- use that information as part of their decision-making process, or
- communicate their decision by talking, using sign language or by any other means.

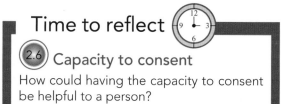

Time to reflect

2.6 Capacity to consent

How could having the capacity to consent be helpful to a person?

If someone makes a decision about treatment that most people would consider to be irrational, it does not constitute a lack of capacity if the person making the decision understands the reality of their situation.

For example, a person who refuses to have a blood transfusion because it is against their religious beliefs would not be thought to lack capacity. This is because they understand the reality of their situation and the consequences of their actions.

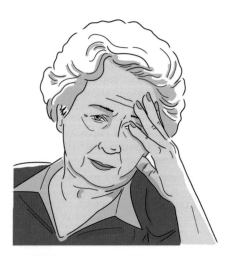

Figure 3.4 **Choice**

However, someone with anorexia (an eating disorder) who is severely malnourished yet rejects treatment because they refuse to accept that there is anything wrong with them would be considered incapable. This is because they do not understand the reality of their situation.

Research and investigate

2.6 Finding out about which aspects of treatments might be refused

Try to find out what other aspects of treatments might be refused.

Changes in capacity

Your capacity to consent can change. For example, you may have the capacity to make some decisions but not others, or your capacity may come and go.

In some cases, people can be considered capable of deciding some aspects of their treatment but not others. For example, a person with severe learning difficulties may be capable of deciding on their day-to-day treatment, but incapable of understanding the complexities of their long-term treatment.

Some people with certain health conditions may have periods when they are capable and periods when they are incapable. For example, a person with schizophrenia may have periods when they are considered capable, but they may also have psychotic episodes (when they cannot distinguish between reality and fantasy), during which they are not considered capable.

Capacity can also be temporarily affected by:

- shock
- panic
- fatigue (extreme tiredness)
- medication.

If a person specifically states in their advance decision that they do not want to undergo a particular treatment, this is legally binding. The only exception may be if that person is being held under the Mental Health Act (1983). This is an Act that allows some people with mental health problems to be compulsorily detained in a psychiatric hospital.

Evidence activity

2.6 Explaining what is meant by informed consent

Prepare a leaflet explaining to relatives and carers what informed consent is.

2.7 # Explain own role in the advance care planning process

Staff have different responsibilities and competences relating to particular types of decisions that need to be made during general care planning.

Sometimes it will be necessary to consult with colleagues or other involved parties such as families, carers or advocates. This is to ensure that a person with capacity is provided with accurate information and appropriate support to maximise their ability to take part in the planning process, to weigh-up any risks and benefits and to make decisions.

Staff must be clear about the scope and responsibilities of their own role and the lines of accountability for the person's care. They should recognise when to call for support or assistance from other team members and should consider consulting colleagues from health, social care, or voluntary sector services who may have information or knowledge about the person, which can help in the delivery of safe, effective and timely care.

They should always consult the person concerned, as well as that person's usual carers and people who are close to the person, where the person agrees that this may be done, or the staff member judges that the person has lost capacity to make a specific decision and it is necessary to do so in order to establish that person's best interests.

Sometimes care decisions which become necessary during care delivery will involve complex issues or have major consequences, or be associated with disagreements about the person's capacity to decide. In these circumstances, staff must call on colleagues with appropriate specialist expertise.

- It is therefore necessary that staff develop a good knowledge of access and referral processes within their locality and area of work.
- The person's usual carers and people close to the person may have knowledge or insight to contribute.
- These issues about recognising different responsibilities and competences are also of relevance in considering advance care planning.

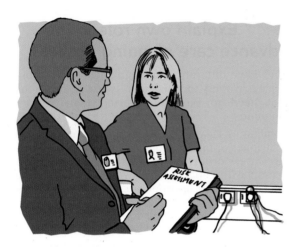

Figure 3.5 Assessing risks

Evidence activity

 Communicating effectively with others in the care planning process

How do you ensure you communicate effectively with others involved in the care planning process? What should you do? What should you not do?

 ### Identify how an advance care plan can change over time

Any record should be subject to review and, if necessary, revision and it should be clear when this is planned. Review may be instigated by the individual or care provider, can be part of regular review or may be triggered by a change in circumstances.

You must make a record of the discussion and of the decisions made. You should make sure that a record of the advance care plan is made available to the person, and is shared with others involved in their care (provided that the person agrees), so that everyone is clear about what has been agreed. If a person makes an advance refusal of treatment, you should encourage them to share this information with those close to them, with other doctors, and with key health and social care staff involved in their care.

You must bear in mind that advance care plans need to be reviewed and updated as the person's situation or views change.

Research and investigate

2.8 **Finding out about why an advance care plan needs to be reviewed**

Find out why an advance care plan needs to be reviewed.

In planning ahead, some people worry that they will be unreasonably denied certain interventions towards the end of their life, and they may wish to make an advance request for those treatments. Some people who are approaching the last days of life may have specific reasons for wanting to receive a treatment which has some prospects for prolonging their life, even if only for a very short time. Some people may hold strong views about receiving clinically assisted nutrition and hydration towards the end of their life, because they see these not as medical treatment but part of basic care.

Evidence activity

 A case study approach to identifying how the needs of an individual who cannot participate in decision making may change over a period of time

Develop a case study identifying a person who cannot participate in decision making. How may their needs change over a period of time?

2.9 Outline the principles of record keeping in advance care planning

Statement of wishes and preferences

This is a summary term embracing a range of written and/or recorded oral expressions, by which people can, if they wish, write down or tell people about their wishes or preferences in relation to future treatment and care, or explain their feelings, beliefs and values that govern how they make decisions. They may cover medical and non-medical matters. They are not legally binding but should be used when determining a person's best interests in the event they lose capacity to make those decisions.

Documentation of advance care planning

There is no set format for making a record of advance care planning discussions, although having a person's wishes documented will prove helpful to those involved in their future care. Professionals who support a person in advance care planning should try to avoid following a rigid prescriptive method of interview and recording of discussions; this can be achieved by using an open question style of dialogue.

Assessment records may be shared with any other member of staff providing health or social care for the named individual, following the principles of 'role-based access', that is, assessors should share with another professional only as much as that person needs to know to play their part in the individual's care. Consent should be sought from the individual being assessed for their records to be shared. In instances where the individual does not give consent, the assessor should discuss with the individual the possible effect this may have on their care and the alternatives available to them. Generally speaking, the 'assessment summary' should be shared between multi-professional teams and across agencies as required, subject to the individual's consent. A copy of this assessment summary should also be given to the individual.

If the person agrees for their record to be shared, it should be ensured that systems are in place to enable sharing between health and social care professionals involved in the care of the person, including out-of-hours providers and ambulance services.

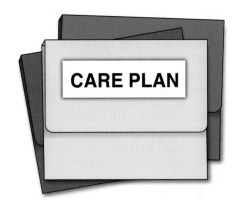

Figure 3.6 Informed consent

Time to reflect

2.9 The importance of maintaining accurate records

Why is it important that accurate records are maintained?

Principles of record making in advance care planning

Healthcare professionals cannot make a record of the discussion without the permission of the individual.

The individual concerned must check and agree the content of the record.

Information cannot be shared with anyone, unless the individual concerned has agreed to disclosure. Where the individual refuses to share information with certain individuals, the options should be explained to them and the consequences made clear.

Any record should be subject to review and, if necessary, revision and it should be clear when this is planned. Review may be instigated by the individual or care provider, can be part of regular review or may be triggered by a change in circumstances.

A clear record of who has copies of the document will help facilitate future updating and review.

Copies in notes should be updated when an individual makes any changes.

Where an advance decision is recorded, it should follow guidance available in the Code of Practice for the MCA and be recorded on a separate document to that used for ACP (http://www.dca.gov.uk/menincap/legis.htm#codeofpractice)

The professional making the record of an advance decision must be competent to complete the process.

Where this is part of a professional's role, competence-based training needs to be available and accessed.

If the individual agrees for their record to be shared, it should be ensured that systems are in place to enable sharing between health and social care professionals involved in the care of the individual, including out-of-hours providers and ambulance services.

For an individual who has lost capacity, disclosure of a statement will be based on best interests.

There should be locally agreed policies about where the document is kept. For example, it may be decided that a copy should be given to the individual and a copy placed in the notes.

Evidence activity

 Read through some notes made in your setting

Read through some notes made in your setting. Do they comply with the principles discussed?

2.10 Describe circumstances when you can share details of the advance care plan

Information cannot be shared with anyone, unless the individual concerned has agreed to disclosure. Where the individual refuses to share information with certain individuals the options should be explained to them and the consequences made clear.

Any record should be subject to review and, if necessary, revision and it should be clear when this is planned. Review may be instigated by the individual or care provider; it can be part of regular review or may be triggered by a change in circumstances.

You must make a record of the discussion and of the decisions made. You should make sure that a record of the advance care plan is made available to the person and is shared with others involved in their care (provided that the patient agrees), so that everyone is clear about what has been agreed. If a person makes an advance refusal of treatment, you should encourage them to share this information with those close to them, with other doctors, and with key health and social care staff involved in their care.

Traditionally, the English common law has protected an individual's right to expect that personal information about him or her will be kept confidential. Information will be protected if it has 'the necessary quality of confidence about it' and has been imparted in circumstances importing an obligation of confidence. For example, information given to a doctor, social worker or lawyer would normally be considered to have this quality of confidence, but a conversation with a friend would not. A duty of confidentiality may also arise as a result of a contract where one party agrees to keep confidential information provided by the other party.

A court can prevent the disclosure of confidential information by injunction and, where appropriate, award damages if unlawful disclosure has been made.

There are two main exceptions to the duty of confidence. Firstly, public interest can override the duty. For example, a psychiatrist could pass on information about a patient to the police if it was felt that the patient was a danger to third parties. Secondly, disclosure of confidential information may be permitted or required by statute or court order.

Evidence activity

 Sharing details of an advance care plan

Provide two examples of when you might need to pass on information relating to an advance care plan.

Following Lord Darzi's review of the NHS in 2008, which included end of life care as one of the eight clinical pathways, the government published the ten-year 'End of Life Care Strategy' for England. The aim is to provide people approaching the end of life with more choice about where they would like to live and die. The strategy covers all adults with advanced, progressive illnesses and care given in all settings. Hospices will play a key role in the implementation of the strategy.

LO3 Understand the person-centred approach to advance care planning

3.1 **Describe the factors that an individual might consider when planning their advance care plan**

Care should be person-centred, meaning that care is focused on the individual to ensure that independence and autonomy are promoted. When planning support, the social care practitioner should use a variety of different methods to collect information about an individual's unique qualities, abilities, interests and preferences, as well as their needs. This means asking the individual what support or service they would like to meet their needs. The social care worker should not make any decisions or start delivering a service without discussion and consultation with the individual involved.

Person-centred care aims to treat the individual holistically as a whole person and not just an illness, and to recognise that all individuals have a right to respect, and be treated with dignity and consideration of their wishes, regardless of their illness. Usually the term person-centred care is linked with the care of people with dementia. However, its principles can be applied to anyone with a life-limiting illness. Historically, a person's illness or condition was at the centre of care, upon which treatment and care plans were based. End of life care adopts the principles of a person-centred approach, thus placing the needs and feelings of the person at the centre, around which everything else is based.

Everybody is different and will experience and respond to illness differently. Therefore, if care staff concentrate on the illness rather than the person behind it, they will be unable to meet the principles of end of life care.

Research and investigate

3.1 **Find out about the key outcomes of Lord Darzi's review**

What were the key outcomes of Lord Darzi's review?

Enabling a care plan to be developed that covers the whole person will make it easier for staff to see beyond the illness, to the person before they became ill. To be able to do this, the care staff will need to consider the individual's biography and identity.

Autonomy and choice over healthcare decisions are major features within the field of end of life care. The advance care planning process allows individuals to exercise control over their end of life care and can provide a number of benefits for the person nearing the end of their life. For example, advance care planning ensures the individual can:

- express their priorities, which can be considered at a future time
- identify where they wish to die
- identify issues which they feel need to be dealt with sooner rather than later
- make professionals aware of their wishes
- where appropriate, promote important discussions between family members
- reduce the risk of conflicting decisions later in the care process.

Key terms

Autonomy is the condition or quality of being autonomous or independent.

In addition, everyone deserves the best quality of care when they are faced with life-limiting conditions and death. Involving service users and giving them control over their end of life care will also ensure they receive care which is person centred and dignified in approach. It is essential that the individual and the people who matter to them are actively involved in decisions concerning their end of life care.

An individual's wishes and preferences will be unique to them. It is essential to use a whole-person approach to assessment and explore the physical, psychological, social, spiritual, cultural and environmental wishes and preferences of each service user. Unrealistic requests should be dealt with sensitively, and possible acceptable alternatives discussed.

Recording and communicating

Once an individual has made their wishes and preferences known, a statement of their wishes will need to be made. Methods of communicating this could be in writing or through recorded conversations. The statement could contain both medical and non medical information, for example:

- preferred place of care
- beliefs and values
- religious needs
- organ donation
- treatment options.

Health and social care workers cannot make a record of the discussion without the permission of the service user. Once the information is recorded, the individual must check and agree the content of the record. Consent to share the advance care plan with anybody else, including the service user's family and health or social care professionals, must be obtained before any information can be shared.

Use your communication skills to:

- Communicate with a range of people on a range of matters in a form that is appropriate to them and the situation.
- Develop and maintain communication with people about difficult and complex matters or situations related to supportive and palliative care.
- Present information in a range of formats, including written and verbal, as appropriate to the circumstances.
- Listen to individuals, their families and friends about their concerns related to supportive and palliative care and provide information and support.

- Work with individuals, their families and friends in a sensitive and flexible manner, demonstrating awareness of the impact of a cancer diagnosis, and recognising that their priorities and ability to communicate may vary over time.

Empathy is the ability to project yourself into the feelings of another person or situation, and is a way of helping people to see a solution to their own problems. Being able to empathise, or identify with a person's material or emotional situation, is necessary for anyone who wishes to attain competence in the skills of counselling, as is the need to understand the basic principles of communication. A carer must practise attentiveness as well as displaying good listening skills, and be able to respond well, saying the right things in the right way. Body language should be used and understood such as, for example, nodding your head a lot, and changing your facial expressions.

Key terms

Empathy means understanding and imaginatively entering into another person's feelings.

Empathy can be demonstrated by using good non-verbal communication. For instance, appearance, facial and eye expressions, the way you sit and stand, the way you use gestures and touch, and the tone of voice that you use.

Good listening requires:

- interest
- the willingness to give time
- respect for the individual
- confidentiality
- the ability to look people in the eye without staring
- restraint:
  - by not finishing words or sentences for people
  - by not interrupting people.

Time to reflect

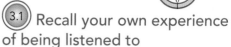

3.1 Recall your own experience of being listened to

When has a person really listened to you? How did this feel? What did they do?

Skills associated with empathy are:

- the ability to communicate your understanding
- to be aware of the tone and manner that you use
- to be aware of your body language
- to resist offering any solutions to problems
- the ability to summarise, which will show people that they have been understood
- the ability to encourage people to talk about problems if they wish to
- giving the person permission to express their feelings
- not judging or criticising individuals
- showing warmth and care for individuals.

Time to reflect

(3.1) The needs and priorities of a person with a hearing impairment

You are supporting a person with a hearing impairment. How can you assess their needs and priorities effectively? Write a short account of the actions you might need to take and why.

You should also acquire the skill of asking open-ended questions. They are questions beginning with 'how', 'who', 'why', 'what', 'where' and 'when' – which cannot be given a 'yes' or 'no' answer, hence encouraging an individual to communicate.

Obviously, the full range of counselling skills and their methods of use require a great deal of training and practice to master, and only some of the basic skills and qualities required by a counsellor and the principles of problem solving are mentioned here. Variations on the forms of counselling provided may be necessary. For instance, if an individual is distressed because of the lack of family visits or because they are feeling anxious about their ill health or prognosis, then facilitating problem solving may be an appropriate course of action. In cases of bereavement or loss, then active listening may be needed. Frequently, counselling may require the merging of different methods, in order to assist the individual with solving their problems and allowing them at the same time to express their fears and thoughts relating to the problem. A good counsellor should be able to recognise which method or methods are appropriate.

Using counselling and listening skills involves maintaining the delicate balance between the use of assertive and responsive behaviour, compared to the negative traits of aggressive and passive behaviour. If the carer's attitude becomes over-assertive, verging on aggressiveness, then the individual's reaction is likely to be either aggressive or passive. On the other hand, if the carer's responsiveness (listening, showing interest, nodding, empathising, summarising what has been said) verges on passiveness (looking uninterested, as if you are not listening), then the same reactions can be expected. A good counsellor should be able to communicate they are listening without interrupting, and be able to feel and show interest in the individual's problems without getting so involved that they cannot counsel properly and effectively. Discrimination, prejudice and judgements should never be involved in counselling, as individuals should be respected for who they are.

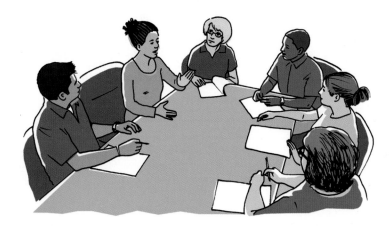

Figure 3.7 **Effective communication**

The role of the counsellor is not to give advice, guidance or information, which are all aspects of helping that can lead to counselling, but are not counselling as such. The counsellor's role is to help somebody to look at a problem in such a way that they can explore it and, therefore, discover ways and means of living more resourcefully and with greater satisfaction. At the end of such a 'helping talk', the individual should be in a better position emotionally than they were at the beginning of the talk. Counselling is therefore talking with a purpose and with a goal, not just 'letting off steam'. 'Letting off steam' produces a lot of energy, and if this energy can be directed into more positive action and attitudes, then counselling will have taken place.

The role of the worker in supporting the counsellor is to help assess if the individual needs counselling; they may do so by monitoring the individual and consulting other members of the care team, communicating with the individual about the purpose of counselling and just what is involved, accessing the services of a counsellor, supporting individuals before, during and after counselling, if necessary, and to give the counsellor any appropriate support or information.

Power relationships

The central role of communication is establishing rapport and a therapeutic relationship, and this requires health and social care professionals to adapt communication approaches to meet the cultural needs of patients in a non-threatening manner. Incorrect perceptions of roles and power can hinder effective support and communication. The individual who speaks a different language may need communication approaches that meet their cultural expectations and needs. The 'doctor knows best' syndrome can create an unhealthy dependency, and now the general trend is more in favour of patient–partnership working and sharing information, evaluation and responsibility. Individuals usually want to be more involved and more active in their decision making.

Evidence activity

3.1 Explain why you need to involve the person you are providing care for in all decision making and the consequences if you do not do this

Think about why it is important to ensure the person you are providing care for is involved in all decision making. What could be the consequences if they are not involved?

3.2 Explain the importance of respecting the values and beliefs that impact on the choices of the individual

It must be acknowledged that individuals' values may differ, and what is considered acceptable to one person may be unacceptable to another.

These values may be influenced by a number of factors including our life experiences, culture, race or religion. For example, most women would find being examined by a male doctor acceptable. However, certain religions, or indeed individuals, may find this completely unacceptable and not allow this to take place. All care workers should be sensitive to the personal beliefs and wishes of others, even if they are different to their own. Negotiation and compromise may be possible; if not, then reporting to a senior colleague is recommended.

The right to choose

We all expect that we have a right to choose. Being cared for does not alter this right. A person does not lose all ability to do things for themselves or make choices just because they become 'a client'/'patient'/'service user'. It is important to maintain a person's chosen daily activities, maintain their physical activities and keep the body exercised in the following ways:

- Mentally – it keeps the mind alert
- Emotionally – it provides stimulation, interest, a sense of self-esteem and individuality.
- Socially – it keeps contact with others and maintains social skills and identity.

Activities where the individual can make choices may include:

- Choosing recreational activities
- Choosing diet and fluids
- Having visitors
- Having a say in how the care setting is organised and the care they receive
- Choosing hygiene facilities and standards
- Choosing to care themselves
- Communicating using their preferred method and language.

Care workers can show respect and preserve dignity by always supporting individuals' choices and upholding their rights, being polite, patient and helpful. An abrupt, impatient or intolerant attitude will humiliate and dehumanise the individual and should be considered abusive. Care settings where care practices are institutionalised do not maintain dignity, privacy or show respect.

Supporting individual's choices

Privacy may be viewed as privacy of information, the provision of private areas for individuals and privacy that involves covering the body. All individuals have the right to be provided with a private area to wash, dress, attend to toilet needs, meet with visitors, receive treatment, relax or be alone. Clothing should be of the person's choice and should cover the body adequately to maintain dignity. People should also be offered advice and support to choose clothing appropriate for their personal needs and the activities they are undertaking. Other care activities where support for individual's choice can be given could include:

- The individual being supported to choose their own toiletries and personal grooming items

- Promotion of self-management skills – supporting the individual to do what they are able for themselves
- Providing aids and equipment to enable the individual to meet their needs, e.g. with hygiene and mobility
- Supporting the individual's preferences with regard to personal hygiene methods
- Ensuring means of calling for assistance are available to the individual
- Promptly attending to the individual's requests for assistance.

It is very important that you show respect for people who are not well. This can be achieved in a number of ways. Together these will help to maintain a person's self esteem, build confidence and encourage independence.

Evidence activity

3.2 Supporting an individual's choices

Nerissa has limited speech. How can you ensure you and other staff are fully aware of Nerissa's wishes and preferences?

3.3 Identify how the needs of others may need to be taken into account when planning advance care

All carers, whether they provide, or intend to provide, regular and/or substantial amounts of care, have the right to have their views and requirements taken into account when considering how they should make provision to a person accessing services. Holistic care planning is a process of discussion between patients and their care providers that may or may not include family and friends. Its aim is to understand individuals' preferences to support their end of life experience.

Time to reflect

3.3 Your feelings at a time when your needs were not fully considered or taken into account

When have the needs of your relatives, friends or carers also needed to be considered? How did you feel about this?

Many people, when told they have a life-limiting illness, may feel very frightened and lonely, believing that others do not understand. They may react very differently, some wanting to talk about their diagnosis, others wanting to avoid the subject whilst they come to terms with the way their life is changing. The age of the dying individual may affect how people discuss the death. The death of an elderly person is generally easier to accept than that of a young child.

It is assumed that healthcare staff will be comfortable with death and dying. They are not expected to have difficulties discussing these issues. However, some healthcare staff may feel uncomfortable and do experience difficulty discussing death and dying. This may be because:

- They are new to the post and have not received any training or instruction, therefore lacking knowledge and understanding
- They may not have come to terms with or understand their own attitudes towards death and dying
- They may fear the terminally ill person will blame them or respond in a way that they do not know how to deal with
- They may be afraid or saying the wrong thing and upsetting the individual and their family.

The more comfortable and confident staff are encouraged to feel about death and dying, the more likely they are to understand and, in turn, fulfill people's individual needs and wishes.

A good death

End of life care aspires towards a good death for all people who are diagnosed with a life-threatening illness. Everybody knows they will die one day, but as a rule people who are young, fit and healthy do not think about their own mortality. However, people who have been diagnosed with a life-threatening illness, or those who are old and frail, may be more aware of their own mortality. Many people would feel happier if they knew their affairs were in order and that they weren't leaving it for their family to sort out after their death. Some may wish to plan their own funeral. Many people are afraid that dying will be unpleasant or painful and hope for a 'good death'. Individuals may have different perceptions of a 'good death'. Therefore there is no one definitive explanation of what is meant by a good death. However, a 'good death' may be defined as 'one with dignity, among friends and without pain'. A 'good death' can also be defined as 'peaceful, one without pain, in a place of choice, where physical, emotional, cultural and spiritual needs are met in accordance with the person's wishes'.

Individuals who have been diagnosed with a life-threatening illness may start planning their own death, deciding where they would like to die and who they would like to be present. They may write a living will, detailing what they do and do not want to happen.

A living will is a legal document that is only valid if it is signed and dated. It is up to the individual where they keep it. However, medical staff and family will need to know its whereabouts so they can access it.

It is important for the care staff to be aware of and to respect the individual's cultural and religious beliefs and practices, as this will influence how carers can meet the individual's needs as death approaches and afterwards. If care staff respect the individual's privacy and dignity as well as their culture, beliefs and practices, not only will the individual believe they are having a good death, but the relatives will also observe their loved one having a good death.

A bad death

A 'bad' death may be defined as 'one where the dying person experiences uncontrolled pain and discomfort; lack of acceptance; their needs and wishes are unmet or ignored; staff and carers are unwilling to listen; there is a lack of information; individuals may be afraid or lonely; or death may be sudden and the individual may not have had time to get their affairs in order, or to say good-bye to their family and friends'.

Being open and able to discuss death and dying

Dying is the one certain thing that we know will happen to us, but it is still an emotive issue. It is a subject that is seldom addressed. This may be because we do not know who to discuss it with, or when aspects of our mortality should be raised.

Some individuals will only discuss death and dying when faced with their own mortality. Some individuals are so reluctant to discuss death and dying that they only want to inform family of what they would like to happen following death. Others may be willing to discuss death and dying but be afraid to discuss their own death, for fear of upsetting those close to them. Some may not be able to understand what is happening to them, that is, a child or someone with dementia. It is important for care staff to be aware of their own attitudes towards death and dying, as this will then enable them to feel comfortable enough to discuss it with those who are dying.

Death and dying can be a difficult subject to discuss. Therefore, it is important for care staff to show compassion and sensitivity when discussing such a delicate and personal issue. The more comfortable and confident the care staff, family and friends are encouraged to feel about death and dying, the more likely they are to understand and in turn, fulfill people's individual needs and wishes.

Difficulties faced in discussing death and dying

The period leading up to someone's death and their dying can be a very emotional and frightening time for all involved.

Many people when told they have a life-limiting illness may feel very frightened and lonely, believing that others do not understand. They may react very differently, some wanting to talk about their diagnosis, others wanting to avoid the subject while they come to terms with the way their life is changing. The age of the dying individual may affect how people discuss the death. The death of an elderly person is generally easier to accept than that of a young child. It is assumed that healthcare staff will be comfortable with death and dying. They are not expected to have difficulties discussing death and dying. However, some healthcare staff may feel uncomfortable and do experience difficulty discussing death and dying. This may be because:

- they are new to the post and have not received any training or instruction, therefore lacking knowledge and understanding
- they may not have come to terms with or understand their own attitudes towards death and dying
- they may fear the terminally ill person will blame them or respond in a way they don't know how to deal with
- they may be afraid or saying the wrong thing and upsetting the individual and their family.

The more comfortable and confident staff are encouraged to feel about death and dying, the more likely they are to understand and, in turn, fulfil people's individual needs and wishes.

Supportive care helps the patient and their family to cope with the condition and treatment of it – from pre-diagnosis, through the process of diagnosis and treatment, cure, continuing illness or death and into bereavement. It also helps the patient to maximise the benefits of treatment and to live as well as possible with the effects of the disease. It is given equal priority alongside diagnosis and treatment. Supportive care should be fully integrated with diagnosis and treatment.

It encompasses:

- self-help and support
- user involvement
- information giving
- psychological support
- symptom control
- social support
- rehabilitation
- **complementary therapies**
- spiritual support
- end of life and bereavement care.

(National Council for End of life care 2008 **www.ncpc.org.uk/palliative_care.html**)

> ## Key terms
>
> Complementary therapies: the practice of medicine without the use of drugs; they may involve herbal medicines, self-awareness, biofeedback or acupuncture.

Research and investigate

3.3 Find out why we have such a big taboo about discussing death and dying

Why do we have such a big taboo about discussing death and dying?

3.3 Identifying the needs of others

Prepare a brief information guide stating how the needs of others may need to be taken into account when planning advance care.

End of life care is part of supportive care. It embraces many elements of supportive care. It has been defined by NICE as follows:

> 'End of life care is the active holistic care of patients with advanced progressive illness. Management of pain and other symptoms and provision of psychological, social and spiritual support is paramount. The goal of End of life care is the achievement of the best quality of life for patients and their families. Many aspects of End of life care are also applicable earlier in the course of the illness in conjunction with other treatments.'

End of life care aims to:

- affirm life and regard dying as a normal process
- provide relief from pain and other distressing symptoms
- integrate the psychological and spiritual aspects of patient care
- offer a support system to help patients live as actively as possible until death
- offer a support system to help the family cope during the patient's illness and in their own bereavement.

Therefore, end of life care is really part of supportive care, sharing and embracing many of its elements (National Council for End of Life Care).

The role of healthcare staff in supportive care is not only to support the individuals who are dying and their families, but also the other members of the care team. Terminal care is the care of the person in the last hours, days or weeks of their life and has usually been used with reference to terminal illnesses such as cancers.

The distinction between terminal care and end of life care lies in the fact that end of life care can help at all stages of the illness from diagnosis onwards, while treatment is in progress and at the end of life.

3.4 **Outline what actions may be appropriate when an individual is unable to or does not wish to participate in advance care planning**

The Mental Capacity Act sets out what approach needs to be taken when assessing capacity. The first point is that capacity must be assessed on a decision-by-decision basis. Clearly, somebody who is unconscious will not have capacity. However, it will be the case for many people that they might have capacity to make some decisions, but not others. For example, somebody might have the capacity to decide what they want to wear, eat or drink. They might not have the capacity to make complicated financial decisions about their pension or investments. There is no such thing as a blanket lack of capacity.

That means that you will need to identify the decision that has to be taken. Then you need to assess whether the patient has the capacity to make that decision himself. The Act contains a two-stage test, and a prohibition.

The prohibition is that you must not make judgements about somebody based on superficial appearances. You must not assume that somebody lacks capacity to make a particular decision simply on the basis of their age, their appearance, their condition, or an aspect of their behaviour. Those are factors that can be taken into account, but they are not sufficient of themselves. You must assess each person as an individual. This is a very important aspect of the Act – it is intended to ensure that people are not discriminated against simply because, for example, they are old or live with a particular condition, such as a learning disability or dementia. There is a similar prohibition when it comes to assessing best interests.

Time to reflect

 3.4 Deciding what to do if a person does not want to be involved in their care assessment and planning

What action should you take if a person does not want to be involved in their care assessment and planning?

Once it has been decided that a person does not have the capacity to make a particular decision for himself, somebody else will need to take that decision on their behalf. Unless it is in a situation in which the person has made a valid and applicable advance decision to refuse treatment, whoever makes that decision must make it in the best interests of the person concerned.

The fact that the person does not have capacity to make a particular decision does not mean that they should be ignored or left out of what is going on. Where possible, their views should be obtained, the decision should be explained, and they should be involved in what is happening. The fact that a person does not have the capacity to make a particular decision does not diminish their humanity. They still need to be treated with respect. Quite apart from anything else, doing this may also make it easier to implement the decision that has been made.

Evidence activity

3.4 **Assessing the needs and priorities of a person with dementia**

You are supporting a person with dementia. They view things very differently to that of their carers. How can you assess their needs and priorities effectively? Write a short account of the actions you might need to take and why.

3.5 **Explain how an individual's care or support plan may be affected by an advance care plan**

Personalised care planning empowers individuals, promotes independence and helps people to be more involved in decisions about their care. It centres on listening to individuals, finding out what matters to them and finding out what support they need.

Personalised care planning is essentially about addressing an individual's full range of needs, taking into account their health, personal, family, social, economic, educational, mental health, ethnic and cultural background and circumstances. It recognises that there are other issues, in addition to medical needs, that affect a person's total health and well being. It is therefore a holistic process, treating the person 'as a whole', with a strong focus on helping people, together with their carers, to achieve the outcomes they want for themselves. In doing this, it should open up more choices that are relevant for people with long-term conditions. This is demonstrated well in the delivery of personal health budgets.

Good care planning can make a huge difference to people's lives. It enables individuals with long-term conditions to plan their care, have strategies in place to cope with exacerbations of their condition and have all the relevant information they need to make informed choices and decisions. Supporting people to self-care means they have more confidence and control over their condition and understand how it affects their lives. Individuals with long-term conditions will be at different stages on their journey and their ability to take more control will depend to some extent on what stage of that journey they have reached. Someone who has just been diagnosed with a long-term condition will have different needs to someone who understands and has accepted their condition, or someone requiring end of life support. Depending on the complexity of the person's need, a multidisciplinary team of staff may be involved in the care planning process. As a minimum, a care planning discussion ought to focus on:

- agreeing the individual's goals (e.g. I want to lose weight, stop smoking, get out more, get a job)
- providing information (timely, relevant, ongoing, could be in the form of an Information Prescription)

- supporting individuals to self-care, to take a more active role in their own health
- agreeing on any treatments, medications, or other services such as access to support groups or structured education programmes, e.g. the Expert Patient Programme
- agreeing any actions
- agreeing a review date.

A care plan quite simply records the outcomes from a care planning discussion, including any actions agreed. It could be a written document, an electronic document or both. The person owns the care plan and can share it with carers and other family members if they wish. People with low level or moderate needs may not want a written document; they may prefer to record anything agreed in their patient notes. They may decline a care plan, or not be happy with the term 'care plan', as it may imply the need to be 'cared for' when they have full and active lives. This is why in some areas it is called a health plan or self-management plan.

For those with complex health and social care needs, a care plan is likely to be a more detailed written document, which may also be called a support plan. It is important that people with complex health and social care needs have:

- a lead coordinator such as a community matron or specialist nurse
- a contingency plan for crisis episodes or exacerbations of their condition
- action plans to attain their goals
- a detailed medication plan and date for review.

The most important thing is that the discussion has taken place, that outcomes are recorded in an agreed format and that people know they have a plan to manage their condition.

Time to reflect

(3.5) **Accurately recording all decisions made and the wishes of the person**

What is the importance of accurately recording all decisions made and the wishes of the person?

What are the benefits of a care plan?

The overarching aim of care planning and agreeing a care plan is to improve the quality of care and outcomes for people with a long-term condition by engaging them more in decisions about their care and to take control of their own health. This process is the central thread of long-term conditions management. Planning care in this way is more proactive and meets people's full range of needs.

For example, overcoming anxiety and depression that was previously undiagnosed means a person can have better health outcomes and be less likely to need repeated GP appointments or emergency admissions. Similarly, crisis planning and knowing whom to contact can reduce unplanned admissions; self-managing can slow progression of disease. This benefits individuals and NHS staff and organisations through improved quality of care, increased job satisfaction and efficiency savings.

How do multiple care plans feed into an overarching care plan?

A person may have one or several treatment/management plans. For example, they may have been referred to a physiotherapist for a special assessment to agree a self-care plan; they may also have agreed a health plan with, for example, a weight loss clinic.

These documents should feed into an overarching care plan, providing additional information about aspects of their overall care package to be shared with the people who are involved in contributing towards that person's care.

It is recommended that it become common practice for all healthcare staff who have contact with a person to refer to their overarching care plan to check that the care they are agreeing supports that person's stated goals.

The role of the healthcare professional in care planning

Supporting people to manage their health and their condition better by taking them through a process of discussion, shared decision making and ongoing support as part of the care planning approach enables healthcare professionals to work in a more inclusive way – working with people rather than doing to them.

Good communication skills are crucial for optimising a care planning discussion and supporting individuals to self-care. It is vital that healthcare professionals have the right skills, approaches and behaviours to deliver high-quality personalised services for individuals with long-term conditions.

Preparing others

As well as thinking about how to approach a care planning discussion, preparing the individual for the appointment is also beneficial; for example, with prompts about which questions to ask, by sending them copies of letters to other clinicians about them or sharing test results with an explanation of what they mean. Encouraging individuals to get the most out of a discussion and to really have an expectation that they can ask what they want and that they are equal partners in the discussion is core to personalised care planning.

> ### Evidence activity
>
> **Person-centred planning**
>
> Why is person-centred planning so important? How can you ensure it is fully implemented at all times?

Assessment summary

Your reading of this chapter and completion of the activities will have prepared you to demonstrate your learning and understanding of end of life care. To achieve this unit, your assessor will require you to:

Learning outcomes	Assessment criteria
Learning outcome **1**: Understand the principles of advance care planning by:	(1.1) describing the difference between a care or support plan and an advance care plan See Evidence activity 1.1, p.54
	(1.2) explaining the purpose of advance care planning See Evidence activity 1.2, p.56
	(1.3) identifying the national, local and organisational agreed ways of working for advance care planning See Evidence activity 1.3, p.57
	(1.4) explaining the legal position of an advance care plan. See Evidence activity 1.4, p.57
	(1.5) explaining what is involved in an 'Advance Decision to Refuse Treatment' See Evidence activity 1.5, p.59
	(1.6) explaining what is meant by a 'Do Not Attempt Cardiopulmonary Resuscitation' (DNACPR) order See Evidence activity 1.6, p.60

Learning outcome **2**: Understand the process of advance care planning by:	explaining when advance care planning may be introduced See Evidence activity 2.1, p.61
	outlining who might be involved in the advance care planning process See Evidence activity 2.2, p.62
	describing the type of information an individual may need to enable them to make informed decisions See Evidence activity 2.3, p.64
	explaining how to use legislation to support decision-making about the capacity of an individual to take part in advance care planning See Evidence activity 2.4, p.65
	explaining how the individual's capacity to discuss advance care planning may influence their role in the process See Evidence activity 2.5, p.65
	explaining the meaning of informed consent See Evidence activity 2.6, p.67
	explaining own role in the advance care planning process See Evidence activity 2.7, p.68
	identifying how an advance care plan can change over time See Evidence activity 2.8, p.68
	outlining the principles of record keeping in advance care planning See Evidence activity 2.9, p.70
	describing circumstances when you can share details of the advance care plan See Evidence activity 2.10, p.70

Learning outcomes	Assessment criteria
Learning outcome **3**: Understand the person-centred approach to advance care planning by:	(3.1) describing the factors that an individual might consider when planning their advance care plan See Evidence activity 3.1, p.74
	(3.2) explaining the importance of reflecting the values and beliefs that impact on the choices of the individual See Evidence activity 3.2, p.75
	(3.3) identifying how the needs of others may need to be taken into account when planning advance care See Evidence activity 3.3, p.78
	(3.4) outlining what actions may be appropriate when an individual is unable to or does not wish to participate in advance care planning See Evidence activity 3.4, p.79
	(3.5) explaining how an individual's care or support plan may be affected by an advance care plan See Evidence activity 3.5, p.81

Good luck!

Web links

Alzheimer's Society	www.alzheimers.org.uk
Care Quality Commission (CQC)	www.cqc.org.uk
Cruse Bereavement Care	www.crusebereavementcare.org.uk
Department of Health	www.dh.gov.uk
Huntington's Disease Association	www.hda.org.uk
Macmillan Cancer Support	www.macmillan.org.uk
Marie Curie Cancer Care	www.mariecurie.org.uk
Multiple Sclerosis Society	www.mssociety.org.uk
National Council for Palliative Care	www.ncpc.org.uk
National End of Life Care Programme	www.endoflifecareforadults.nhs.uk
Parkinson's Disease Society	www.parkinsons.org.uk
The Motor Neurone Disease Association	www.mndassociation.org
Princess Royal Trust for Carers	www.carers.org

4

For Unit EOL 304
Support the spiritual well-being of individuals

What are you finding out?

End of life care is about caring for people who have an advanced, progressive and incurable illness so they can live as well as possible until they die. It is about providing support that meets the needs of both the person who is dying and the people close to them.

Spirituality is important to patients and families. Spiritual care is increasingly identified as an integral part of healthcare systems across the world, and this is particularly so in palliative and end of life care where a holistic approach is established as both a philosophy and model of care.

The reading and activities in this chapter will help you to:

• Understand the importance of spirituality

• Understand how to assess the spiritual needs of a person

• Understand the impact of values and beliefs on own and others' spiritual well-being.

LO1 Understand the importance of spirituality for individuals

 Outline different ways in which spirituality can be defined

Spirituality is not religion and is not even necessarily affiliated with religion. While the definition of spirituality is different for everyone, there are some common themes associated with spirituality:

- the idea of a process or journey of self-discovery and of learning not only who you are, but who you want to be
- the challenge of reaching beyond your current limits; this can include keeping an open mind, questioning current beliefs, or trying to better understand others' beliefs
- a connectedness to yourself and to others: spirituality is personal, but it is also rooted in being connected with others and with the world around you. This connection can facilitate you finding 'your place in the world'
- meaning, purpose, and direction: spirituality, while it doesn't necessarily solve or reach conclusions, often embraces the concept of searching and moving forward in finding the meaning, purpose, and direction for your life
- a higher power, whether rooted in a religion, nature, or some kind of unknown essence.

■ Research and investigate

(1.1) Defining spirituality

Write your own definition of what you think spirituality is.

Evidence activity

(1.1) Sam

Sam has just been admitted to your setting and wants to discuss spirituality with you. Devise a list of the points you think Sam might want to include in the discussion.

 Define the difference between spirituality and religion

Spirituality is whatever gives a person meaning, value and worth in their life. This may not necessarily be an organised religion or god. It is the strength and solace people gain from things that are important to them that give a person a purpose to living. It may be the love of their family, the peace of the countryside or enjoying creating a piece of art.

■ Research and investigate

(1.2) Find out about one religion and list its key points

Investigate one religion and list its key points.

Even though many people consider spirituality to have the same meaning as religion, the terms differ. Religion is a system of faith and worship with a reverence to a power commonly described as 'god'. Spirituality is much less formal and constitutes anything which provides an individual with some meaning and understanding of life.

Evidence activity

(1.2) Spirituality and religion

List the guidance and support you think a person can derive from a) spirituality and b) religion.

 Describe different aspects of spirituality

Spirituality extends beyond an expression of religion or practice of religion. There is a pursuit for a spiritual dimension that not only inspires, but creates harmony with the universe. That relationship between ourselves and something greater compels us to seek answers about the infinite. During times of intense emotional, mental, or physical stress, man searches for transcendent meaning, frequently through nature, music, the arts, or a set of philosophical beliefs. This often results in a broad set of principles that involves more than all religions.

Research and investigate

(1.3) Find out about the different aspects of spirituality

What do you think are the different aspects of spirituality?

While spirituality and religion remain different, sometimes the terms are used interchangeably. This lack of clarity in their definitions frequently leads to debates. Suppose one's spirituality leads to the formation of a religion? Is it necessary for a spiritual person to be religious? Through certain actions, an individual may appear outwardly religious, and yet lack any underlying principles of spirituality. In its broadest sense, spirituality may include religion for some, but still stands alone without a connection to any specific faith. The search for spirituality sends us wandering down paths that offer unsatisfactory results. The Far East offers shrines that contain hundreds of statues. Worshippers choose a statue that most resembles an ancestor and pray to it. A piece of stone or rock represents one's personal and intimate relationship with the spiritual realm. During the fourth and fifth centuries BC, Athens was a vital culture centre with a world-famous university. The Athenians were firm and rigid in their spirituality as well as their reverencing of their deities (i.e. religion).

Evidence activity

(1.3) Explain the differences between two approaches to expressing spirituality

Investigate two ways in which spirituality is expressed and explain the differences between the two approaches.

(1.4) Explain how spirituality is an individual experience

Spirituality will mean different things for people. Generally, the term spirituality refers to an individual's sense of meaning and purpose; for example, lots of people will ask questions at some point in their lives such as 'Why are we here?' and 'What is our purpose?' Spirituality refers to the exploration of an individual's 'inner-self' or 'higher-power'.

Many people think spirituality is focused solely on religion; however, religion is often only a minor part of spirituality and, if you're not religious, you can still explore your spirituality without any reference to religion. Inner-peace and fulfilment are often terms associated with spirituality, as the concept focuses on listening to your 'inner-self' and your true desires.

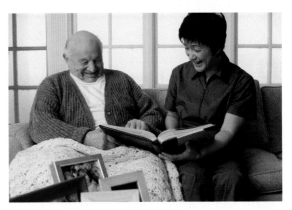

Figure 4.1 Inner peace and fulfilment are often associated with spirituality

Time to reflect

(1.4) Differing views on spirituality

Do people have different views on spirituality and what it means to them? Why might this be so?

Often, individuals will want to explore their spirituality if they feel they haven't yet found what's important to them in life. They may have lots of money, a nice house, a great job and an expensive car, but they may still experience an inner empty, numb feeling. In today's world it's easy to lose sight of what's important and to simply live life day to day without really looking deeply at whom we truly are and what will bring real meaning into our lives.

Spirituality concentrates on exploring our inner wants and desires and can totally transform some people's lives, offering them a sense of contentment and meaning. Enlightenment is also a term used in relation to spirituality and can be defined as 'recognition of a meaning to existence that transcends one's immediate circumstances'. Exploring spirituality is a unique experience for each individual, and how deeply you want to explore is completely up to you.

Key terms

Identity is the fact of being whom or what a person or thing is.

Evidence activity

1.4 Respecting a person's view on spirituality

Explain how you can respect a person's view on spirituality.

Time to reflect

1.5 List key aspects of your identity

What is your identity? List key aspects.

1.5 Explain how spirituality defines an individual's identity

Grief felt for the loss of a loved one, the loss of a treasured possession, or a loss associated with an important life change occurs across all ages and cultures. However, the role that cultural heritage plays in an individual's experience of grief and mourning is not well understood. Attitudes, beliefs, and practices regarding death must be described according to myths and mysteries surrounding death within different cultures.

A person's identity is tied to their spiritual and cultural beliefs. So it is just as important to meet these needs as it is to meet physical and psychological needs. Recognising each person's unique individuality is vital. Healthcare staff have a responsibility to meet the whole care needs of the individual, including the spiritual and cultural aspects. This can be achieved in a number of ways, including:

- appreciating that everyone has a spiritual dimension; almost everyone has something that makes life worth living
- recognising that some people will have a religious and/or cultural element to their spirituality
- practising active listening
- being mindful of one's non-verbal messages
- appreciating that people will express their spirituality and possible spiritual pain in different ways
- acknowledging that there may be conflicts within families around spiritual issues.

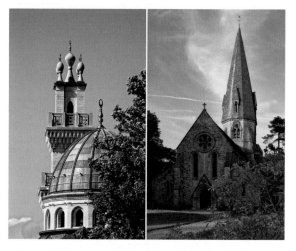

Figure 4.2 A person's identity is linked to their spiritual and cultural beliefs

Meeting a person's cultural needs can be achieved by:

- treating each person as an individual
- learning from the person – ask the person and their family about their culture and specific rituals, beliefs and traditions
- researching the different cultural groups within the healthcare setting – find out what information is available within your care setting; speak with managers and colleagues who may be excellent sources of information
- being sensitive to a person's past – as this may have an effect on the way the person behaves and reacts to your support
- understanding what values different cultures hold with regard to illness and the administering of care and treatment – this will determine how willing they are to accept help and treatment from others

- reassuring the family that professionals will support, not replace, their role
- providing clear, understandable information in a form that is user friendly.

Key terms

Values are important and enduring beliefs or ideals shared by the members of a culture about what is good or desirable and what is not.

Research and investigate

(1.5) Planning or providing for a person to meet their religious or spiritual needs

What can you plan or provide for a person to meet their religious or spiritual needs?

Individual, personal experiences of grief are similar in different cultures. This is true even though different cultures have various mourning ceremonies, traditions, and behaviours to express grief. Helping families cope with the death of a loved one includes showing respect for the family's cultural heritage and encouraging them to decide how to honour the death. Important questions that should be asked of people who are dealing with the loss of a loved one include:

- What are the cultural rituals for coping with dying, the deceased person's body, the final arrangements for the body, and honouring the death?
- What are the family's beliefs about what happens after death?
- What do the family feel is a normal expression of grief and acceptance of the loss?
- What does the family consider to be the roles of each family member in handling the death?
- Are certain types of death less acceptable (e.g. suicide), or are certain types of death especially hard to handle for that culture (e.g. the death of a child)?

Death, grief, and mourning spare no one and are normal life events. All cultures have developed ways to cope with death. Interfering with these practices may interfere with the necessary grieving processes. Understanding different cultures'

response to death can help physicians to recognise the grieving process in patients of other cultures.

Evidence activity

(1.5) Supporting religious or spiritual needs

Find out about which people or organisations you can ask for support and guidance on meeting religious or spiritual needs.

Which other people or organisations can you ask for support and guidance on meeting religious or spiritual needs?

(1.6) Outline the links between spirituality, faith and religion

Spirituality is a term that has been used in many arenas and carries a range of meanings. It is difficult to define and is more often described by saying what it is not.

The phrase 'body, mind and spirit' singles out spirit as a part of being human and shows it as different to both thinking and the physical being, which can include the emotions. Spirituality is often used to describe people's higher aims, which spring from a deep understanding of who they are.

People in some faiths see spirituality as being linked to a higher 'being' outside of ourselves, which is transcendental – for example, God, Allah or Yahweh. People in other faiths describe this spirit as existing in the cosmos and seek union with it – for example, the process of enlightenment in Buddhism – while others, such as Hindus, worship one god, aspects of which are expressed through multiple deities.

There is also the view that spirituality has nothing to do with a transcendental being but stems from within a person. Humanists have argued for a broader approach to spirituality where this aspect of being human exists in the lives of all people, whether they believe in a god, have no view of God, or resist religious doctrines and practice.

Research and investigate

(1.6) Personhood

Find out what 'personhood' means.

As the word 'spirituality' carries such confusion, many people have tried to come up with a new word that is infused with positive aspirations, meaning and power, without the negative dimension that causes separation and division. However, expressions such as 'well-being', 'personhood' and others are limited in different ways; so, however imperfect the word 'spirituality' may seem, it still has value in describing something special. One way to get around this is to agree on a working definition whenever the word is used.

Spirituality is an important part of being human. Learning and developing our own spirituality involves developing a capacity to reflect and connect with the world. It is about making sense of our lives and understanding the story of how we fit with ourselves, others and our environment. There is a struggle to define outcomes from spiritual journeying, but the challenge for practitioners is to find sympathetic ways of describing spiritual progress, rather than to abandon supporting it because it is hard to measure.

Faith usually relates to the main world religions: Judaism, Islam, Christianity, Buddhism, Hinduism and Sikhism. There are other faiths that also have their own theologies and practices. Each religion can also have different denominations and approaches that bring a range of practices and experiences for members.

Evidence activity

 1.6 Make a list of world religions

Make a list of world religions. You will be surprised how many there are!

 1.7

Explain how an individual's current exploration of spirituality may be affected by their previous experience of spirituality, faith or religion

There will be some people who already have a rich experience of faith and religion, some who may have no formal experience but have a deep understanding of their own humanity and some who have perhaps had more negative experiences of spirituality or religion.

People grow up in different traditions of religion. For some people, spiritual beliefs are at the centre of their understanding of life. For others, religion influences the cultural traditions that they celebrate; for example, many Europeans celebrate Christmas even though they might not see themselves as practising Christians. Discrimination can take place when people assume that their customs or beliefs should apply to everyone else.

Research and investigate

1.7 Your views about spirituality

Since working in the sector have your views about spirituality changed? If so, why have they changed?

Some experts warn that religious beliefs can be harmful when they encourage excessive guilt, fear, and lowered self-worth. Similarly, practitioners should avoid advocating for particular spiritual practices; this can be inappropriate, intrusive, and induce a feeling of guilt or even harm if the implication is that ill health is a result of insufficient faith. It is also important to note that spirituality does not guarantee health. Finally, there is the risk that people may substitute prayer for medical care or that spiritual practice could delay the receipt of necessary medical treatment.

Religious experience (sometimes known as a spiritual experience, sacred experience, or mystical experience) is a subjective experience, in which an individual reports contact with a transcendent reality, an encounter or union with the divine.

A religious experience is most commonly known as an occurrence that is uncommon in the sense that it doesn't fit in with the norm of everyday activities and life experiences, and its connection is with the individual's perception of the divine. Studying religious experience objectively is a difficult task, as it is entirely a subjective phenomenon. However, commonalities and differences between religious experiences have enabled scholars to categorise them for academic study.

Many religious and mystical traditions see religious experiences as real encounters with God or gods, or real contact with other realities, while some hold that religious experience is an evolved feature of the human brain that is amenable to normal scientific study.

Spirituality and religion are usually positive and helpful to people, but they can sometimes take an unhelpful turn and be destructive rather than integrative.

Evidence activity

1.7 Jessie

Jessie is a Christian but has been put off religion and spirituality since her diagnosis of leukaemia. Why have Jessie's views changed?

LO2 Be able to assess the spiritual needs of an individual

2.1 Support the individual to identify their spiritual needs and how and by whom these can be addressed

As people approach the end of their lives, they and their families commonly face tasks and decisions that include a broad array of choices, ranging from simple to extremely complex. They may be practical, psychosocial, spiritual, legal, existential, or medical in nature. For example, dying persons and their families are faced with choices about what kind of caregiver help they want or need, and whether to receive care at home, or in an institutional treatment setting. Dying persons may have to make choices about the desired degree of family involvement in caregiving and decision making. They frequently make legal decisions about wills, advance directives, and Durable Powers of Attorney. They may make choices about how to expend their limited time and energy. Some may want to reflect on the meaning of life, and some may decide to do a final life review or to deal with psychologically unfinished business. Some may want to participate in planning rituals before or after death. In some religious traditions, confession of sins, preparation to 'meet one's maker', or asking forgiveness from those who may have been wronged can be part of end of life concerns. In other cultural traditions, planning or even discussing death is considered inappropriate, uncaring, and even dangerous, as it is viewed as inviting death.

All end of life choices and medical decisions have complex **psychosocial** components, ramifications, and consequences that have a significant impact on suffering and the quality of living and dying. However, the medical end of life decisions are often the most challenging for terminally ill people and those who care about them. Each of these decisions should ideally be considered in terms of the relief of suffering and the values and beliefs of the dying individual and their family. In addition, any system of medical care has its own primary values that may, or may not, coincide with the values of the person. For example, in most western medical systems the principles of individual autonomy (though not to the exclusion of family members and intimates) and informed consent are primary. In contrast, many cultures eschew the principle of autonomy and the principle of interactive, community decision making is thought to be the ideal. Therefore, well-intentioned presentations of treatment or care possibilities by healthcare providers may overlook a particular person's wish not to discuss death.

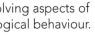

Key terms

Psychosocial means involving aspects of both social and psychological behaviour.

Time to reflect

2.1 Discussing your spiritual needs

With whom would you wish to discuss your spiritual needs?

When someone is admitted to a hospital or care setting, their faith/beliefs, religious or spiritual practices and relationship with their family and community will be of vital importance to them. It is impossible to know all of the intricacies of specific religious and spiritual belief systems. What is more important is treating individuals seriously and humanely; and trying to understand and support the issues each individual faces and the challenges they are grappling with. Chaplaincy services are there to provide specialist advice, support and services; and also, importantly, to liaise with faith communities in the wider society. It is important to increase mutual understanding and trust within the multidisciplinary team so as to respond to the spiritual needs of people and promote a positive culture.

Evidence activity

2.1 Adele

Adele has discussed her spiritual needs with you. Who can help you to meet Adele's needs?

2.2 Identify how an individual's emphasis on spirituality may vary at different stages of their life experience

Serious illness can have a disorientating and depersonalising effect on a patient, leaving them feeling vulnerable or powerless as events and suffering overtake them. In hospitals or other care settings, it is often nursing staff or carers who are presented with the signs of spiritual distress, so the ability to recognise this is essential in order to support the patient as meaningfully as possible.

Spiritual distress may manifest itself in a variety of ways. Some patients are very articulate about the origin of their feelings, while others may be unaware or sceptical about the potential emotional or spiritual dimension to their experience of illness. It is important to remember that relatives and friends will also be affected by what is happening and are likely to be suffering in their own way. They may also exhibit signs of spiritual distress and therefore need support too.

The events and pace of change during serious illness and deteriorating health can feel overwhelming for patients and their families. Clear communication and information at each step can help patients to understand how their illness is affecting them and what can be done to help. It is also important to offer enough information so that patients can maintain some sense of control over choices and decisions that are open to them and are able to make plans for themselves or their family.

Family and those close to the patient may find it difficult to know how to discuss the implications of the patient's condition or potentially distressing topics. They are likely to welcome the opportunity to ask questions about the illness, what to expect and, perhaps, how to respond to questions that the patient is asking them. As long as the patient is happy for information about their illness to be shared, discussion of these issues may enable relatives to understand the dying process as they accompany their loved one. It is important to explain that the nature of the care has changed and that the main purpose is now to ensure a comfortable, peaceful and dignified death, as far as this is possible. They should be encouraged to continue talking together as family and friends as openly as they feel able to, as this is likely to provide mutual comfort and support.

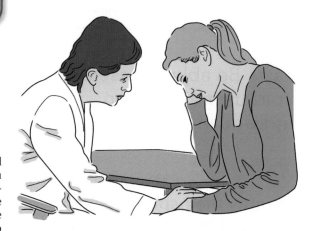

Figure 4.3 Serious illness can have a disorientating and depersonalising effect

Research and investigate

2.2 Explore why a person's emphasis on spirituality may change throughout their lifetime

Why would a person's emphasis on spirituality change throughout their lifetime?

Ethical issues may arise in relation to the care of those nearing death. In all medical care the most important ethical requirement is respect for the patient. Respecting the patient implies respecting the good of the patient's life, however long or short this may be. It also implies that the patient should be involved in discussions and decisions about their care and treatment. Wherever possible these decisions should be in keeping with the patient's wishes, values and beliefs. Where they are known, it is helpful to record these within the general care plan or as part of an advanced care plan. Treatment or care decisions should not be made on behalf of a competent patient without their consent.

Evidence activity

 2.2 Provide an explanation of ethics and their impact on end of life care

Explain what ethics are and how they impact on end of life care.

■ Research and investigate

 2.3 Explain your understanding of a timeline and how to prepare one

What is a timeline and how would you start preparing one?

2.3 ■ **Take action to ensure that the individual's spiritual well-being is recognised appropriately in their care plan**

If our spirituality and identity come under pressure, this can threaten our very existence. In an initial assessment it won't be possible, or even appropriate, to discover everything about an individual, but it will be important to ascertain, if possible, what the framework is for their:

- internal world
- external world.

For a very isolated person, their most important relationship may be with a place, an animal, or a friendly neighbour or shopkeeper. For someone with a religious faith, prayer times, meditation, the opportunity for 'sacred' or other space, diet or connection with the faith community and priest, imam, rabbi, etc. will be essential.

Another approach to mapping spirituality and identity might be to follow a timeline:

- **Setting the scene**: what is life all about? Issues of belief (not necessarily religious), meaning, value and purpose.
- **The past**: experiences, especially around loss, and loss of trust. What creates resilience or openings of anxiety and fear for the future?
- **The present**: what is the current situation and are there ways that the individual and their experiences can be attended to positively? Is there space for recovery and growth?
- **The future**: hopes, aspirations and plans. Working in partnership.
- **Remedies**: drawing on the individual's own coping mechanisms as much as possible, including the mutuality of support.

Other important aspects to spirituality and identity could be:

- **Identity**: what are the components which make up an individual's identity; nature and nurture, ethnicity, values, and belief systems? How has that identity travelled and could it still be developing?
- **Love and relationships**: how does the individual relate to those intimate with them? Are there fractured relationships which need healing?
- **Vocation and obligation**: what sense of calling and obligation does the person have in their life?
- **Experience and emotion**: how does this experience of illness and the associated feelings relate to the individual's life meaning? How are 'negative' feelings handled?
- **Courage and growth**: how has the individual coped with crises in the past and how might they summon up courage for the future?
- **Reciprocity**: what can the individual give, and have the potential to give others?
- **Gifts:** what talents, skills and creativity does the individual have?

The results of this spiritual assessment should be incorporated into the care plan.

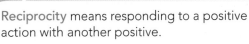

Key terms

Reciprocity means responding to a positive action with another positive.

Care should be person-centred, meaning that care is focused on the individual to ensure that independence and autonomy are promoted.

When planning support the social care practitioner should use a variety of different methods to collect information about an individual's unique qualities, abilities, interests and preferences as well as their needs. This means asking the individual what support or service they would like to meet their needs. The social care worker should not make any decisions or start delivering a service without discussion and consultation with the individual involved.

Once a plan has been produced, it should be viewed as a working document, which can be changed and adapted according to the changing needs of the individual. Careful thought is required as to how care is to be delivered.

A spiritual organisation is one with an awareness of its deeper values, identity and aspirations. These are apparent in the building it occupies, in its leadership, among its staff, in its reputation in the community and among the people who access its services.

The integrated nature of these factors is a key feature of a spiritual organisation and can be seen at all levels of the organisation, from strategic management at board level to the relationships between the workers and the people using services.

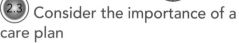

Time to reflect

 2.3 Consider the importance of a care plan

What is the importance of a care plan?

By virtue of their relationship to the patient, it is also important to include close family or carers in significant discussions and decisions, unless the patient does not wish to involve them. This is particularly important if the patient is no longer competent to make their own decisions. There are occasions when there may be differing views or conflict between the patient and family, creating an ethical dilemma about how to meet their respective wishes. Clinical staff have a professional responsibility to consider the patient as their primary concern and may need to find other ways to support the family, possibly through spiritual or counselling care. As a patient is nearing death, they are increasingly unlikely to respond to many medical interventions. It is therefore important to ensure that treatment decisions, including decisions to withdraw treatment, are based on accurate diagnosis of the cause of deterioration and regular reassessment,

as it is unethical to burden a patient with treatment that is futile. In this situation, the priorities of care shift towards maintaining good symptom relief and providing palliative care.

Evidence activity

 2.3 Kaplan

Kaplan's care plan has just been reviewed, but it does not contain any information about his spiritual well-being. Explain the action you should take and why.

LO3 Understand the impact of values and beliefs on own and an individual's spiritual well-being

3.1 Analyse how your own values and beliefs may impact on others when communicating about the individual's spiritual well-being

A worker who is comfortable with their own spirituality will be able to allow this exploration and expression from a firm base of respect and worth. If extreme views are shared, these can be explored within a context of open listening and calm debate.

Time to reflect

 3.1 Your own values and beliefs

Take some time to reflect on your own values and beliefs.

Anyone who works in health and social care needs to be secure in their own spirituality and their sense of self, in order to hear a range of views and maintain a safe space where these can be explored with mutual respect. More positively, a worker with a secure sense of their own spirituality can bring deeper understandings into their work and offer explorations to people at a level beyond merely learning skills and changing behaviour, thus giving a more integrated, holistic approach.

Evidence activity

 Explain the importance of being aware of your own values and beliefs as a worker and how they could impact on other people

Explain why it is so important that you, as a worker in the sector, are aware of your own values and beliefs. How could they impact on other people? How do you think past ways of working may affect present ways of working?

3.2 Identify how the values and beliefs of others may impact on the individual

3.3 Identify the effects on own values and beliefs when meeting the spiritual needs of individuals and others

One of the most important things to remember when meeting the spiritual needs of others is not to assume that another person has the same values, beliefs, and practices that you do. Use your observation, listening, and questioning skills to learn what is important to the other person and how they see the world. Be open to learning about other ways of seeing and living in the world.

Spirituality is often seen as a broader concept than religion. Some spiritual beliefs are particular to an individual, whereas the beliefs attached to a religion are shared by large groups of people who follow established teaching.

People express their spirituality in many different ways and spiritual beliefs can influence the decisions that service users make about the treatment they receive or how they want to be supported. Giving service users the space to lead full spiritual lives requires staff to be sensitive to cultural difference.

Time to reflect

3.3 Your values and beliefs and how they impact on your daily life

How do your values and beliefs impact on your daily life?

Talking about spirituality may touch something very personal in you, as well as in people accessing services. However helpful talking may be, it can also be difficult. This difficulty should not stop you helping people to express their spirituality, because for many of them it will be central to their existence.

You cannot consider the spirituality of service users without thinking about your own. Understanding your own beliefs and values and acknowledging their importance to you can help you to understand and respect the key role that service users' spirituality may play in their identity, and how it influences the way that they cope with their current problems.

Evidence activity

 Ask two people about their values and beliefs and explain how they differ

If possible ask two people about their values and beliefs. How do they differ?

LO4 Be able to support individuals' spiritual well-being

4.1 Access resources and information to support the individual's spiritual well-being

Wherever you work – managed care, the hospital, rehabilitation, long-term care unit, home health care, or any of the multiple settings that make up our vast healthcare system – you are probably caring for patients that are more culturally diverse than ever before.

In a multicultural society, such as Great Britain, there are many citizens from various religions and cultural groups who have different belief systems and traditions in relation to death. It is important to be aware of these differences, as you may well be required to support an individual in the planning, preparation or implementation of some aspects.

In order to provide safe, quality and cost-effective care for diverse cultures, healthcare professionals need to strive to achieve cultural competence. The term 'cultural competence' is used to describe people and organisations that work effectively with their own culture and with cultural groups different from their own. It involves a set of attitudes, practices, behaviours and policies that enable a person, agency, or system to work effectively in multiethnic, pluralistic, and linguistically diverse communities.

One area most affected by our struggle with cultural diversity is in effective treatment of pain. Cultural background has long been recognised as a major influence in how one perceives and reacts to painful situations. Pain has both personal and cultural meanings. Although patients may experience a similar condition or surgical procedure, pain response may differ dramatically.

Research and investigate

 4.1 Find out about the resources your setting accesses to support spiritual well-being

Which resources does your setting access to support spiritual well-being?

The ability of healthcare professionals to break through cultural barriers is key to providing effective pain management in patients that are culturally diverse. The ethnicity and culture of the healthcare team may be as important as the patient's culture in determining the impact of pain and how it is treated.

Pain is a subjective and universal experience that individuals of all ages and every culture experience. Pain is not a concrete entity, but is often treated this way and without a holistic approach by all members of the interdisciplinary team. In order to understand pain, the common phrase used to define pain is that 'pain is whatever the experiencing person says it is, existing whenever the experiencing person says it does'.

When treating a patient from a different culture, the patient's concern for symptoms must be treated with as much concern as the actual physical symptoms that are present. Because people attribute meaning to their pain, patients attempt to order the experience of their pain, and what it means to them and those close to them, through personal narratives of their illness. These stories are not fixed, but constantly told and retold. There is a sense in which the narratives not only reflect the pain experience, but also create it. Key metaphors and rhetorical devices appear to be chosen by the patient as a way to make sense of the pain experience.

Nursing, medical, and hospital cultures influence pain assessment, decision making, and care. An understanding of the impact of culture on the pain experience is crucial to effective care. There are individual and cultural differences in terms of pain management. Some patients may want constant pain medication, while others will stoically deny the need for any pain medication. The role of the healthcare provider is to help patients advocate for what feels appropriate for them within their cultural context. Understanding the patient may be difficult when patients are from different cultures and speak languages disparate from that of the healthcare provider. The responsible healthcare professional seeks out staff members, as well as family or friends, with whom the dying patient can communicate. Patients should be allowed to freely express their questions and/or fears about their impending deaths even when such conversations are uncomfortable for the professional.

It is often best to anticipate a patient's pain needs, since cultural or religious reasons may inhibit a patient from requesting pain medication even when it is medically necessary for recovery. Also, not every patient will share a desire for the least intrusive medication possible. When alternatives are available, it is best to check with the patient; which forms would they prefer?

Evidence activity

 4.1 Kaitlin

Kaitlin is Muslim. Explain the information and resources you can access to support Kaitlin's spiritual well-being.

Contribute to the creation of an environment that enables individuals to express aspects of their spiritual well-being

Spirituality, like other qualities, is not 'either present or absent'. The issue is more a case of to what degree it is present, rather than whether it is there at all. The level of spirituality can be increased by identifying sensitive practices and building on these to improve the quality of spirituality. It can be increased by people celebrating it in small everyday things as well as through large events. When a staff team wants to seriously address increasing its sensitivity and spirituality, it is able to build attitudes, behaviour and processes into the organisation's culture.

One of the reasons people feel uncomfortable about spirituality is that it sits outside the main part of their work and is seen as an 'add-on'. As spirituality is about integrity it defeats its object if it is separate and different to the other things that a project does. Rather than seeing spirituality as distinct, it can be integrated into all aspects of the work.

Time to reflect

4.2 Review your work environment and consider whether it enables people to express their spiritual well-being

Review the environment you work in; do you think it enables people to express their spiritual well-being?

Principles and values describe the kind of attitude towards care you would appreciate if you were being cared for yourself. Creating a positive care environment requires health and social care workers to adopt principles and values, which become a 'way of being and working'. Principles and values include recognising and acknowledging the following points:

- empowerment of individuals
- promotion of choice
- promotion of rights (to dignity and privacy, safety and security)
- recognition of preferences

- involvement of individuals in planning their support
- respect for diversity, including individual identity, cultural beliefs, moral beliefs and values
- anti-discriminatory practice
- maintaining confidentiality.

Evidence activity

4.2 Explain how to create an environment that supports a diverse range of needs in terms of spiritual well-being

People accessing your service have diverse needs in terms of their spiritual well-being. How can you create an environment which supports a range of needs?

4.3 Support the individual to take opportunities to explore and express themselves in ways that support their spiritual well-being

Effective communication requires that the right conversations take place by staff with the right skills at the right time. It is important that they recognise and respond to the signs that someone is approaching the end of life and help them to start planning their future care. Staff need to create early and repeated opportunities for people to talk about these issues. They should be guided by the person on timing, pace and content, and respect the wishes of those who do not wish to discuss such matters.

When communicating with individuals it is important that you give them your full attention. This will ensure that you and they are able to communicate effectively, that any barriers and difficulties are identified, and strategies put in place to meet individuals' needs.

It is very important to interpret the needs of individuals and to motivate them to communicate. The way in which you approach individuals, and your willingness to help, will create an atmosphere in which they feel relaxed and able to communicate. Patience is essential, as people will feel uncomfortable if they are aware of being rushed, or feel that you are becoming impatient when they are trying to communicate. Provide them with alternative methods to assist communication, and seek the advice and support of key people within and outside your care organisation to provide extra support.

While encouraging people to communicate, you must remember that people should never be forced into communicating. They should be free to choose the use of gestures, symbols, drawing and the written word if they wish, providing this does not interfere with therapy or progress.

Some people may not wish to communicate at all. This may be due to a specific communication difficulty or a psychological or emotional reason. This should be reported so that the person can be referred for assessment by specialists.

Evidence activity

 Changes or adaptations to communication that could be used to ensure you are aware of a person's priorities

4.3

What changes or adaptations to communication might you need to utilise to ensure you are aware of a person's priorities?

4.4 Support the individual to participate in their chosen activities to support their spiritual well-being

Person-centred care is about providing care and support that is centred or focused on the individual and their needs. We are all individual and just because two people have the same medical condition, for example, dementia, it doesn't mean that they require the same care and support. You will need to develop a clear understanding about the individuals you are working with. This includes their needs, their culture, their means of communication, their likes and dislikes, their family and other professionals' involvement so you can promote and provide person-centred care and support. Person-centred values provide a foundation on which you can base and build your practice. You need to understand what the values are, how you can promote them and why they are important. A value is simply what is important in the life of the person you are supporting.

Time to reflect

4.4 Important aspects of communication when supporting people to take part in activities

What aspects of communication are important when supporting people to take part in activities?

Patients or their relatives sometimes ask for particular things to be done or incorporated into care during the last days of the patient's life. It is important to be sensitive to such requests. Something that might seem unimportant to an onlooker can be of great importance to the patient. It might be a personal item with deep sentimental value, or a religious item such as a crucifix, a rosary or a prayer book. Holding and touching such items may be the only prayer that a patient has the energy to make. Seeing such items at a patient's bedside is also a further indication of their spiritual and religious needs and should prompt carers to ask questions about them and encourage patients to talk about their beliefs.

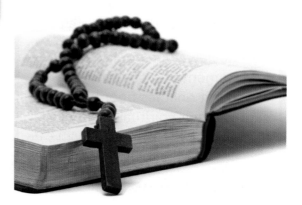

Figure 4.4 Carers should encourage patients to talk about their beliefs

Evidence activity

 Design an activity plan to meet the spiritual well-being of a person who is Greek Orthodox

Design an activity plan for a person to meet their spiritual well-being. The person is Greek Orthodox.

4.5 Access any additional expertise required to meet the individual's spiritual needs

Everyone, whether religious or not, needs support systems, especially in times of crisis. Many patients, carers and staff, especially those confronting serious or life threatening illness or injury, have spiritual needs and welcome spiritual care. They face ultimate questions of life and death. They search for meaning in the experience of illness. They look for help to cope with their illness and with suffering, loss, fear, loneliness, anxiety, uncertainty, impairment, despair, anger and guilt. They conjure with the ethical dilemmas which advancing technology and heightened expectations generate at the beginning and end of life. They address in depth, perhaps for the first time, the realities of their human condition. Those actively associated with a faith community, now statistically in a minority, expect to derive help and comfort from their religious faith and from the faith communities to which they belong. The beliefs and rituals of their religion and the ministry of its leaders and members are often sufficient to meet their spiritual needs. On the other hand, the majority who have no such religious associations, yet recognise their need for spiritual care, look for a skilled and sensitive listener who has time to be with them. That is, a person who will acknowledge the deep desires and stirrings of their spirit, recognise the significance of their relationships, value them and take them seriously; a person who can help them to find their inner resources to cope with their difficulties and the capacity to make positive use of their experience of illness and injury. The care or support service must offer both spiritual and religious care with equal skill and enthusiasm.

Time to reflect

4.5 Your spiritual well-being

Who supports you to meet your spiritual well-being?

In some healthcare settings, spiritual care may not readily be offered on a one-to-one basis, for example, to those with severe communication difficulties, but rather by the creation of a communal spirituality and a positive spiritual environment in which patients are well cared for and staff find fulfilment in their work. Responsibility for this rests primarily with management and staff. The role of the spiritual caregiver in such units is to offer support to staff and carers as may be needed.

Evidence activity

4.5 Practitioners accessed in your service

Review the practitioners accessed in your service. Are there unmet needs? If so, which practitioners could support these?

4.6 Outline the benefits of working in partnership with faith and non-religious communities to support the needs and preferences of the individual

There has been an increased emphasis on different health and social care agencies and the community working together in partnership. This includes sharing good practice and contributing to the support of people accessing services. For example, when supporting children and families the social worker and the health visitor need to work together, using their different qualities and skills to develop a support plan.

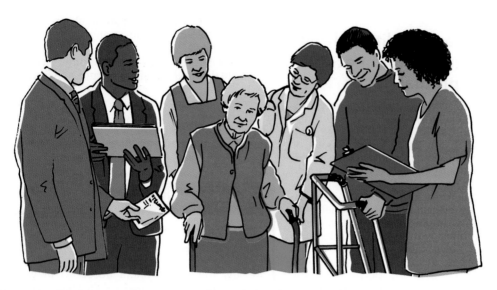

Figure 4.5 Working together in partnership includes sharing good practice and contributing to the support of people accessing services

Multidisciplinary working is about teams of workers from different specialist professions and services working together, in order to prevent problems from occurring in the support planning process. Effective multidisciplinary working may mean that the individual who is receiving care gets a better service and a better outcome from service providers. Working well with other agencies allows for all the different options to be considered, and resources can be offered for inclusion in a support plan. In this way, realistic expectations and the limits of what can be offered can be discussed by all the different agencies, the support plan manager and the individual who is going to receive care services. A well organised multidisciplinary team can help avoid duplication of roles and conflicts of responsibilities. However, working with different professionals and organisations can prove challenging, as each professional may have different priorities, which can involve allocation of financial and other resources. Key staff within the team may have different approaches to the targets and goals that have been set. For example, the worker could have a task-centred approach, just focusing on the specific task they have been asked to undertake and ignoring the wider picture. The social worker may have very different priorities, which could be linked to funding of services. The funding might not be adequate to meet all the needs of the individual named in the support plan. There could also be problems with acknowledging differences in opinions about how the rights and needs of the individual should be met, which could add to conflicts within the team.

Research and investigate

 Partnerships in your organisation

What partnerships exist in your organisation?

Evidence activity

 Services provided by the faith communities in your area

Explore the faith communities in your area. What services do they provide? Prepare a leaflet showing what provision is available.

NORTHBROOK COLLEGE SUSSEX
LEARNING RESOURCE CENTRE
LIBRARY

Assessment summary

Your reading of this chapter and completion of the activities will have prepared you to demonstrate your learning and understanding of end of life care. To achieve this unit, your assessor will require you to:

Learning outcomes	Assessment criteria
Learning outcome **1**: Understand the importance of spirituality for individuals by:	**1.1** outlining different ways in which spirituality can be defined See Evidence activity 1.1, p.86
	1.2 defining the difference between spirituality and religion See Evidence activity 1.2, p.86
	1.3 describing different aspects of spirituality See Evidence activity 1.3, p.87
	1.4 explaining how spirituality is an individual experience See Evidence activity 1.4, p.88
	1.5 explaining how spirituality defines an individual's identity See Evidence activity 1.5, p.89
	1.6 outlining the links between spirituality, faith and religion See Evidence activity 1.6, p.90
	1.7 explaining how an individual's current exploration of spirituality may be affected by their previous experience of spirituality, faith or religion See Evidence activity 1.7, p.91
Learning outcome **2**: Be able to assess the spiritual needs of an individual by:	**2.1** supporting the individual to identify their spiritual needs and how and by whom these can be addressed See Evidence activity 2.1, p.92
	2.2 identifying how an individual's emphasis on spirituality may vary at different stages of their life experience See Evidence activity 2.2, p.92
	2.3 taking action to ensure that the individual's spiritual well-being is recognised appropriately in their care plan See Evidence activity 2.3, p.94

Learning outcomes	Assessment criteria
Learning outcome **3**: Understand the impact of values and beliefs on own and an individual's spiritual well-being by:	(3.1) analysing how your own values and beliefs may impact on others when communicating about the individual's spiritual well-being See Evidence activity 3.1, p.95
	(3.2) identifying how the values and beliefs of others may impact on the individual See Evidence activity 3.2, p.95
	(3.3) identifying the effects on own values and beliefs when meeting the spiritual needs of individuals and others See Evidence activity 3.3, p.95
Learning outcome **4**: Be able to support individuals' spiritual well-being by:	(4.1) accessing resources and information to support the individual's spiritual well-being See Evidence activity 4.1, p.96
	(4.2) contributing to the creation of an environment that enables individuals to express aspects of their spiritual well-being See Evidence activity 4.2, p.97
	(4.3) supporting the individual to take opportunities to explore and express themselves in ways that support their spiritual well-being See Evidence activity 4.3, p .98
	(4.4) supporting the individual to participate in their chosen activities to support their spiritual well-being See Evidence activity 4.4, p.98
	(4.5) accessing any additional expertise required to meet the individual's spiritual needs See Evidence activity 4.5, p.99
	(4.6) outlining the benefits of working in partnership with faith and non-religious communities to support the needs and preferences of the individual See Evidence activity 4.6, p.100

Good luck!

Web links

Alzheimer's Society	www.alzheimers.org.uk
Care Quality Commission (CQC)	www.cqc.org.uk
Cruse Bereavement Care	www.crusebereavementcare.org.uk
Department of Health	www.dh.gov.uk
Huntington's Disease Association	www.hda.org.uk
Macmillan Cancer Support	www.macmillan.org.uk
Marie Curie Cancer Care	www.mariecurie.org.uk
Multiple Sclerosis Society	www.mssociety.org.uk
National Council for Palliative Care	www.ncpc.org.uk
National End of Life Care Programme	www.endoflifecareforadults.nhs.uk
Parkinson's Disease Society	www.parkinsons.org.uk
The Motor Neurone Disease Association	www.mndassociation.org
Princess Royal Trust for Carers	www.carers.org

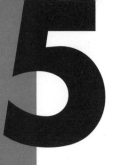

For Unit EOL 305
Supporting individuals with loss and grief before death

What are you finding out?

It is commonly believed that grief is something that is experienced following the death of a loved one, and that the grieving process begins only when the person has died. While in some cases this can be true, in most circumstances grief usually begins before the person dies. When a person is diagnosed with a life-limiting condition, they may begin to experience feelings of loss and grief in relation to the anticipation of death. The person may begin to mourn for themselves and for their own losses. Family and friends may also begin to mourn for the forthcoming loss of their loved one.

Within this chapter you will learn about the impact of loss and grief on individuals approaching the end of life, how you can support these individuals through their experience of loss and grief and how you can manage your own feelings in relation to loss and grief.

The reading and activities in this chapter will help you to:

• Understand the impact of loss and grief on individuals approaching the end of life

• Be able to support individuals through their experience of grief and loss

• Be able to manage own feelings in relation to loss and grief.

LO1 Understand the impact of loss and grief on individuals approaching end of life

1.1 Describe what is meant by loss and grief before reaching end of life

An individual who is diagnosed with a life-limiting condition may begin to experience feelings of loss and grief in relation to the anticipation of death. The person may begin to mourn for themselves and for their own losses. Family and friends may also begin to mourn for the forthcoming loss of their loved one. 'Anticipatory loss' is a term used to describe the sense of loss that occurs before the actual death of a person.

Anticipatory loss forces a person to look at every aspect of their life. The relationship with the person they are losing is examined over and over

again, the closeness of the relationship is analysed in detail and the meaning of the relationship is dissected as the person contemplates their past, present and future. The anticipation of the future, of family events, of future accomplishments are all brought under the spotlight as the person contemplates a life without their loved one in it. These feelings of loss will vary from person to person and may include any combination of the examples in Figure 5.1.

Time to reflect

1.1 What does loss mean to you?
Imagine how you would feel if you received a diagnosis of a life-limiting condition. Make a note of the sorts of losses you might experience following the diagnosis.

The word 'grief' is a term used to describe the emotional reaction that a person may feel in response to loss. Anticipatory grief, also known as preparatory grief, refers to the emotions that a dying

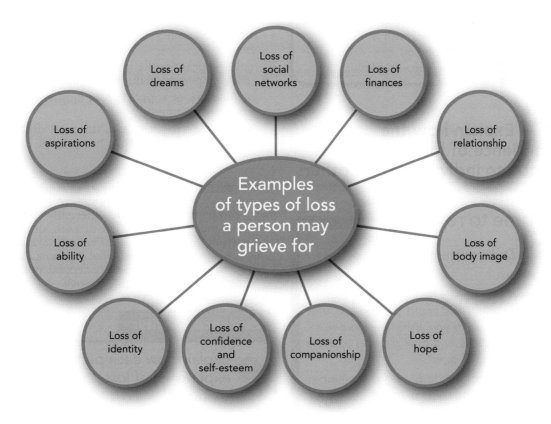

Figure 5.1 'Anticipatory loss'

person may experience on the journey towards the end of their life. The individual's loved ones may also experience anticipatory grief, although not necessarily to the same extent or at the same time. Anticipatory grief is normal. It is an important part of coping with extended illness. Its purpose is to prepare both the person who is dying and their loved ones for the end of life. Unfortunately, it may also be an emotional rollercoaster. Anticipatory grief involves confusing, intense emotions that can swing back and forth. The emotions can become overwhelming and make little sense at all. The feelings of guilt, anxiety and hopelessness can rise to the surface as the person feels a sense of overwhelming helplessness.

Evidence activity

 The meaning of loss and grief before reaching end of life and the types of loss an individual may experience if diagnosed with a life-limiting illness

Describe what is meant by loss and grief before reaching end of life.

Describe the types of loss an individual may experience if diagnosed with a life-limiting illness and how a person can experience grief before reaching the end of their life.

 Explain how the experience of loss and grief is unique to individuals and others

Time to reflect

1.2 Different experiences of loss and grief

Consider a time when you have experienced a loss. This could be any loss that was significant to you. What was your reaction to this loss and how did you express your feelings of grief?

Now ask a colleague or a family member to undertake the same exercise.

Identify any differences which made the experience of loss and grief unique to each of you.

Every individual will experience the concept of death and dying in their own way, and therefore every person's experience of anticipatory loss and grief will be unique to them. This is because we are all individuals with our own unique set of circumstances, and these will shape each person's responses to the experience of loss and grief. There are many factors that can affect an individual's experience of loss and grief, including:

- the age of the person who is grieving – e.g. a child, an adolescent or an adult
- the personality of the person experiencing loss and grief
- the coping skills of the person experiencing loss and grief
- previous life experiences
- the individual's state of health
- the type of relationship the person who is grieving has with the person who is dying – for example, spouse, sibling, parent or friend
- the nature of the relationship with the person who is dying – e.g. close and loving, or remote and troubled
- the way in which the person is facing the end of their life – e.g. if the person is in pain or is restless, or if the person is pain free and at ease
- the grieving person's religious or spiritual beliefs
- cultural practices – e.g. the ways in which the grieving person's culture expresses grief
- availability of support from family, friends and their community
- associated stresses – e.g. financial difficulties, job loss or the breakdown of a relationship.

We can therefore see that not everyone will experience grief in the same way. Even people in the same family, or those who have similar diagnoses and treatments may respond differently to what is happening. Grief is unique to each situation and each individual. It may differ in how long it lasts, how intense it is, and what it means. How, when, and what people grieve is dependent upon so many aspects as highlighted above.

Evidence activity

 Explain how each person's experience of loss and grief is unique

Explain the reasons why people experience loss and grief in different ways.

1.3 Describe stages of loss and grief commonly experienced by individuals with a life-limiting illness

There are different theories regarding the grief process. Most of them differ only in the terminology used and sometimes in the emotions that surface during the different stages of grief. When faced with loss, it is natural for people who are facing death, as well as those they will leave behind, to move through many stages of grief. The grieving process can last for several months or, in some circumstances, much longer. The stages of grief do not necessarily fall into a set order, and they can vary greatly from one individual to another. People may move in and out of these stages at different times throughout the grieving process. Raphael (1984) in *The Anatomy of Bereavement* suggests that the stages of anticipatory grief for both the dying person and those close to the person parallel the stages of bereavement as proposed by Elisabeth Kübler Ross.

These are:

- denial and isolation
- anger
- bargaining
- depression
- acceptance.

It is important to note that not everyone will experience grief in the same way. Some people may not work through the stages in the order in which they are presented here. Sometimes some people will move from one stage to another and some people may miss a stage completely. Some people may get stuck at a stage and may find it difficult to move on. While for some people, the stage of acceptance may help them to come to terms with the fact they are dying, another person may never reach the stage of acceptance.

Stage 1: denial and isolation

The individual may feel numb and bewildered. The person who has received the diagnosis and their family may feel isolated, and may say things such as 'this cannot be true, it isn't happening to me', 'there's been some sort of mistake', or 'the doctor has got the wrong records, I am going to be fine'.

Following the initial shock, the dying person may appear to minimise the seriousness of the diagnosis. This is when the person is expressing denial. Denial is a defence mechanism. The person may attempt to put on a brave face and pretend everything is going to be alright in an attempt to protect others. Even though this phase may last for days, weeks or months, some people may never move beyond this phase.

Stage 2: anger

As the individual begins to come to terms with the reality of what is happening to them, denial often makes way for feelings of intense anger and resentment. Anger is often misdirected and aimed at those around the person, for example, loved ones, or the doctor who gave the diagnosis or even those providing care for the individual. The person may also feel angry with a higher body such as God. It is also common at this stage for the person who is dying to display feelings of resentment or jealousy towards others and question 'Why me?'

Stage 3: bargaining

Eventually the feelings associated with denial and anger start to diminish and this is the time when the individual will start to adjust to the prospect of death. This is the phase where people start to adjust to their goals, hopes and expectations and will start to bargain in order to negotiate deals with themselves, another person or whatever God they believe in. The person may say things like 'Please give me one more chance and I promise I will be a better person'. Loved ones may often go through the same bargaining to negotiate more time with the dying person.

Stage 4: depression

With the realisation that the loss is real and the circumstances cannot be changed, the individual may sink into a deep sadness. The person may feel that nothing matters any more, and may question why they should bother. The person may start to give up hope and may withdraw from making plans for the future. The person may also become less interested in their personal appearance.

Stage 5: acceptance

As long as the individual has had enough time and has been given support in working through the stages of grief, they will reach a stage where they will come to terms with what is happening. This final stage marks the end of the emotional struggle as the individual accepts what will be.

Although the person may have accepted what will be, it is important to note that this is not always a happy time for some people. Although the person may be at peace, their interest in those around them will diminish as they become increasingly weak and tired. The person who is dying may not feel like talking and may show little in the way of enthusiasm for visitors.

Evidence activity

 1.3 Describe stages of loss and grief commonly experienced by individuals with a life-limiting illness

While maintaining confidentiality, undertake a case study to describe how the stages of grief relate to the reactions of a person who has received a diagnosis of a life-limiting illness.

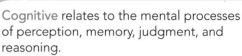 **1.4** # Describe the effects of loss and grief on individuals and others

People respond to and express their experience of loss and grief in their own unique way. The experience of loss and grief can be immensely stressful and can take a great toll on the body, potentially leading to a number of physical, emotional, **cognitive**, behavioural and spiritual manifestations. See Table 5.1.

Key terms

Cognitive relates to the mental processes of perception, memory, judgment, and reasoning.

Table 5.1 Effects of grief on the individual

Physical	Physical effects associated with grief are normal and may include: palpitations, tightness in chest, breathlessness, tightness in throat, headaches, loss of appetite/increased appetite, fatigue, sleep disturbances, hollowness in stomach, dry mouth, lack of energy, weakness of muscles and over-sensitivity to noise.
Emotional	Feelings such as sadness, anger, depression, loneliness, relief and numbness are all common. In addition the individual may also experience feelings of irritability, agitation, restlessness, wanting to be alone, frustration, anxiety, moodiness, guilt, apathy and fear. In some cases the individual may even feel overwhelmed and express an inability to cope. The individual may even express suicidal thoughts.
Cognitive	Disbelief is often the initial cognitive reaction to the news of a loss, especially if the news was unexpected. Although this response is usually temporary, it can persist and lead to denial. Other cognitive effects include feelings of confusion, forgetfulness, difficulty organising thoughts and preoccupation with the prospect of death, which may evoke intrusive thoughts of how the deceased will die or has died.
Behavioural	Although there are a number of behaviours associated with grief which may be of concern to the individual, they generally subside over time. Complications in the grieving process may be indicated if the behaviours impede a person's ability to function. The most commonly reported behaviours include disturbances in sleep, altered appetite, absent mindedness, social withdrawal, vivid dreams, and avoidance behaviour. The person may also use alcohol or other drugs in an attempt to cope with the situation.
Spiritual	The person may respond by questioning their spiritual or religious beliefs. The individual may question or lose their faith. On the other hand, the individual may find solace and comfort through their spiritual beliefs and express their beliefs in a much stronger way than they have done before.

Evidence activity

(1.4) Describe the effects of loss and grief on individuals and others

Using the headings in the table below, describe the possible effects of grief on an individual who is experiencing a loss.

Physical	Emotional	Cognitive	Behavioural	Spiritual

LO2 Be able to support individuals through their experience of loss and grief

(2.1) Support individuals and others to identify the losses they may experience

When an individual and their family are told of a life-limiting illness they may start to grieve in anticipation of the impending loss. As we have already discovered these feelings of loss will vary from person to person and some of them may be secondary to the primary loss. In the initial stage of grief it is common to deny these losses; however, following a period of time, the individual should progress through the various stages of grief, experiencing feelings such as anger and guilt, often leading to feelings associated with depression. Ultimately, the person begins to accept the changed situation and things start to settle down. This all sounds simple within the realms of a text book; however, for the person going through it, this could be a living nightmare. Many people struggle to move through the different stages and become stuck in the denial, anger or depressive stage. Failure to accept the reality of the loss means that the grief cannot been resolved.

Unresolved grief happens mostly as a consequence of denial of the loss. Denial of a loss is an unconscious psychological response against the pain caused by grief. Nobody likes to experience pain, and denial acts to numb the pain associated with loss. The pain is still there, but it is not felt.

When grief remains unresolved, it can lead to other serious problems, including depression, anxiety disorders and even physical illnesses such as heart trouble.

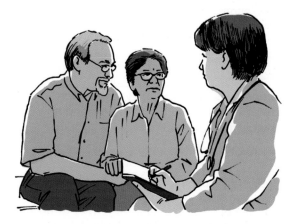

Figure 5.2 Identifying anticipated losses

It is therefore essential that individuals are supported to identify their anticipated losses, in order that they can be supported to come to terms with the full reality of the loss. Acknowledging anticipated loss can enable the person to express and validate their feelings and to identify areas where additional support may be required.

Evidence activity

 Support individuals and others to identify their anticipated losses

Explain how individuals and significant others are supported to identify their anticipated losses within your work environment.

2.2 According to their preferences and wishes, support individuals and others to communicate the losses they may be experiencing

In supporting people to communicate their anticipated losses it is important to realise that people who are grieving value support from caregivers who are friendly, respectful and who treat them as an individual. This can be demonstrated through your manner, your body language, how you say things and your approach to people. Empathy, or trying to put yourself in someone else's shoes, can also help you communicate more effectively.

Key terms

Empathy is about putting yourself in another person's shoes in order to understand how things must feel for the person.

Supporting a person to discuss their anticipated losses can help them to prepare for death, and some people may feel that they wish to do this while they still feel strong enough to express their needs, wishes and preferences.

Below are some ways in which you can support people to communicate their anticipated losses:

- **Give the person time** – this is one of the most important things you can give a person. Demonstrate that you are listening carefully to what they are saying. Avoid interrupting and never try to stop the person from crying. This is a normal part of the healing process.

- **Listen to the person in a non-judgemental and accepting way** – keep your personal thoughts to yourself. The person may need to express a variety of emotions, including crying, swearing, shouting and screaming. It is important to acknowledge these feelings and that they represent how the person is feeling. This is their reality.

- **Avoid distractions and give the person your full attention** – it is important to acknowledge how the person is feeling. It is important to try to put yourself in the person's shoes. Touch can sometimes communicate far more than words. It is also important to acknowledge that touch may be uncomfortable for some people as they may feel it as an invasion of their privacy. It is also important to recognise the boundaries of the relationship as some people experiencing grief can be vulnerable and may misinterpret warmth, compassion and interest.

- **Encourage the individual to discuss their anticipated losses** – it is important that the person is enabled to discuss their anticipated loss as often as they need to. It is important to recognise if the individual is at risk of not being able to move on. If the person appears to be stuck in a phase of grief, for example, denial, he or she may need to be referred for professional support.

- **Recognise that silence is an important part of communication** – don't rush to fill awkward silences with chit chat. Silences are essential and often serve to enable the person to think about what they want to say next.

- **Be familiar with your own feelings about loss and grief** – do not let your own sense of helplessness keep you from reaching out to people who are grieving. Equally do not avoid people who are experiencing loss because you are uncomfortable with discussing their needs. If you have recently experienced a loss yourself, you may not be the best person to provide support for a person who is grieving.

- **Offer reassurance** – reassure the person that their feelings are normal and that the duration of grief can vary from person to person.

- **Do not take anger personally** – anger can be a normal part of the grieving process and it is important to realise that this anger is not directed towards you.

- **Accept that you cannot make the person feel better** – even though you want to make the person feel better it is important to realise that you cannot provide a cure for the person. The individual must work through the process of grief and come to terms with their unique losses.

2.2 Support individuals and others to communicate their anticipated losses according to their preferences and wishes

Explain how you work to support people to communicate their anticipated losses according to their preferences and wishes within your work environment.

2.3 Support the individual through each stage of grief they experience

The first step in supporting a person through the stages of anticipatory grief is to realise that every person is different, with their own set of values and mechanisms for coping. Supporting a person who is nearing the end of their life can be very difficult. It may be difficult to know what to say to the person or to know how to react to the various emotions the person may express.

Table 5.2 Supporting individuals through all stages of grief

Stage of grief	Steps that can be taken to support the individual
Stage 1: denial and isolation	• Give the person time to go over the same ground again and again • Accept the feelings of denial; try not to contradict the person by attempting to make them come to terms with reality • Remain non-judgemental, no matter how critical the person may be of the care they are receiving • Be prepared for extreme swings in mood; these are natural at this stage • Respect that the person may need space and may not wish to talk at this stage • If you or the person are finding talking openly difficult, encourage the person to speak with someone else, for example, their GP or a nurse
Stage 2: anger	• Do not take anger personally; although it may appear to be, it is not directly aimed at you • Acknowledge the validity of the person's feelings. Never ignore or dismiss the person's anger • Encourage the person to discuss their feelings. This is important in order to enable the person to be able to move on to the next stage • Empathise with the person. Try to put yourself in the person's shoes • Ensure you promote choice and independence, as the anger may come from a loss of control • Be understanding and patient • Encourage the person to reflect on their feelings and what helped them to cope with feelings of anger in the past • Let the person know that what they are feeling is acceptable and 'normal'
Stage 3: bargaining	• Encourage the person to talk about their feelings, their hopes and aspirations. Although a person may not be able to hope for recovery, they may still hope for other things and as long as those hopes are realistic, bargaining can help them to maintain a degree of hope • Discuss with the person how they may be able to achieve their hopes and what support may be needed to fulfil their aspirations • Ensure the rest of the care team are made aware of the person's wishes and ensure that any documentation is kept up to date to ensure the person's hopes and aspirations are recorded

Stage of grief	Steps that can be taken to support the individual
Stage 4: depression	• Take time to listen to the person; this is a very important aspect of supporting a person who is suffering from depression • Create an atmosphere which will encourage the person to open up to you; for example, offer the person a cup of tea • Empathise with the person's feelings. Acknowledge the pain the person is feeling, but do not rush in with words of advice • Where appropriate, offer hope. This is very important, as this will help to improve the person's sense of well-being • Respect the person's choices, as not all people will want to talk • Report and document any conversations you have with the individual to facilitate continuity of care
Stage 5: acceptance	• Help loved ones to come to terms with the acceptance, as they may feel rejected, especially if the individual becomes detached from what is going on • Support the person to fulfil any final wishes

Evidence activity

 2.3 Support the individual through each stage of grief they experience

You have been asked to explain to a new member of staff how people are supported at each stage of grief within your work environment. Produce a hand-out to support your explanation.

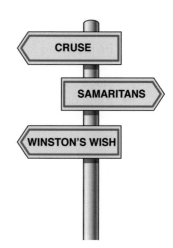

Figure 5.3 Support services

2.4 Support individuals and others experiencing loss and grief to access support services

Although the losses and associated grief that accompanies a life-limiting illness can turn our world upside down, it is something that most people will eventually come to terms with. For those who find loss difficult to accept, it is important that you can reassure them that help is available.

Some people find it useful to talk with other people who have been through similar experiences. Others may find comfort from speaking with a grief counsellor or psychotherapist. It is therefore useful to have some knowledge of organisations that can be contacted if additional support is required. Some examples are given in Table 5.3.

Table 5.3 Examples of some organisations providing support to individuals experiencing loss and grief

Organisation	Services provided
Bereavement Advice Centre www.bereavementadvice.org 0800 634 9494	Provides a free helpline and web-based information service to give information and advice on the many issues and procedures that people are faced with following the death of a person.
British Association for Counselling and Psychotherapy (BACP) www.bacp.co.uk 01455 883300	Provides a nationwide list of local counselling services.
The Compassionate Friends www.tcf.org.uk 08451 232304	TCF is a charitable organisation of bereaved parents, siblings and grandparents dedicated to the support and care of other bereaved parents, siblings, and grandparents who have suffered the death of a child/children.
Cruse Bereavement Care www.crusebereavementcare.org.uk 08444 779400	Cruse Bereavement Care promotes the well-being of bereaved people and enables anyone bereaved by death to understand their grief and cope with their loss. As well as providing free care to all bereaved people, the charity also offers information, support and training services to those who are looking after them.
Institute of Family Therapy www.instituteoffamilytherapy.org.uk 02073 919150	The Institute of Family Therapy provides support for recently bereaved families or those with seriously ill family members.
London Friend www.londonfriend.org.uk 0207 8373337	Provides advice and support for lesbian, gay, bisexual and transgender people following the death of a partner.
Samaritans www.samaritans.org.uk 08457 909090	Provides support for people in times of despair.
Winston's Wish www.winstonswish.org.uk 08452 030405	Provides support for bereaved children and young people.

Research and investigate

(2.4) Bereavement support services

Using any resources available to you, find out what bereavement support services are available in your area and nationally. Put a booklet together detailing all of the sources of support available.

Evidence activity

(2.4) Support individuals and others experiencing loss and grief to access support services

Explain how individuals experiencing loss and grief are supported to access support services within your environment.

LO3 Be able to manage own feelings in relation to loss and grief

(3.1) Describe how own feelings about loss and grief can impact on the support provided

Working in end of life care can be very rewarding. However, we must also acknowledge that it can also be a very stressful and exhausting job. This is because end of life care brings with it a number of unique demands and challenges; for example, health and social care staff very often have to deal with:

- the confrontation of death on a daily basis
- the confrontation of physical and emotional pain on a daily basis
- ongoing establishment and relinquishment of relationships
- demanding and constant care
- grief and sometimes anger expressed by the individual and their families.

When confronted with the unique demands of their work, health and social care staff also have to deal with their own feelings about loss and grief and how these feelings can impact on the care they provide for service users and their families.

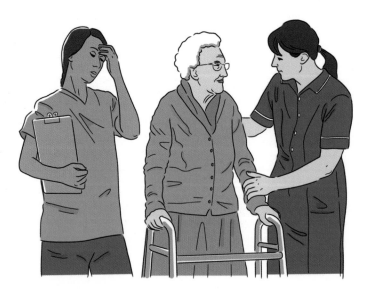

Figure 5.4 Detachment or engagement

It is not just the family and friends who experience loss and grief. There may be times when care staff also experience strong feelings associated with loss and grief, either before or after a person has died. It is important for you to understand that this grief is a natural response to loss and to recognise that it is not unprofessional to show your emotions. In fact, if you do not express this grief, or it is not acknowledged, it could lead to stress-related problems and impact on the quality of care you are able to deliver. Active grieving can therefore help to prevent work related stress and 'burn-out'.

Where health and social care staff are dealing with death on a daily basis, there is a higher risk of something called 'cumulative grief'. This is where unresolved grief from a number of bereavement experiences accumulates, and affects the person in a way which leads to a deep sense of bereavement.

Key terms

Cumulative grief is where unresolved grief from a number of bereavement experiences accumulates and affects the person in a way which leads to a deep sense of bereavement

Working in an environment where death occurs frequently calls for a balance between engagement and detachment, and the balance requires ongoing self-monitoring. If balance is lost, the detachment or engagement can become dysfunctional and this may result in the inability to meet your own needs or the inability to care for others.

Several things may happen if you are unable to maintain a healthy balance in a work environment where death occurs frequently. These may include:

- decreased tolerance or sensitivity – you may be unable to adequately meet the demands of your work
- the tendency to become overly cynical, and your sense of the world may become clouded
- a post-traumatic stress reaction, which could include sensory imprints or flashbacks – sights, sounds, or smells that bring back a certain situation
- difficulty in maintaining hope at work or in your personal life.

It is therefore important for health and social care staff to recognise this type of grief and to seek help from their support network or from a trained counsellor.

Suggestions for coping with grief

Ways in which you may cope with grief include the following:

- Don't be afraid to express your feelings of grief.
- Attend the individual's funeral if you have the opportunity to do so.
- Write a letter of condolence to the family.
- Talk about your feelings with your family, friends and colleagues (remember to maintain confidentiality).
- Talk about your feelings with your manager.
- If you are religious, it may help to remember the person in your prayers.

Evidence activity

3.1 Describe how own feelings about loss and grief can impact on the care you give

Explain the steps you personally take to ensure you deal with your own feelings of loss and grief within your workplace.

Describe how cumulative grief could impact on the care you deliver within your workplace.

3.2 Use support systems to manage own feelings brought on by loss and grief

It is essential that you recognise when you may need support. Observing and listening to the way that members of the care team support individuals may be of help to you.

Care staff should never be made to feel that they are being 'unprofessional' by showing signs of grief. If they hide their grief they are in danger of become 'burnt out', where the stress of dealing with the stressful aspects of end of life care are unsupported, and the person suffers stress, anxiety and loss of motivation which affects their personal and professional life.

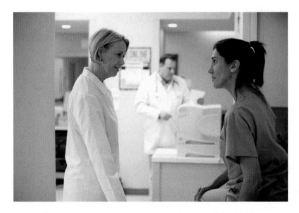

Figure 5.5 Managing your own feelings

There should be provision within your care organisation for staff to discuss and work through their grief. Referral to professional agencies should be available if a staff member is struggling to come to terms with their feelings of loss and grief.

Your feelings may seem unimportant as you support people who are dying and the bereaved on a daily basis. Acknowledging your own grief and stress may make you feel guilty, that it is not you who should feel this way. However, to avoid excess stress and burnout you must look after your own well-being:

- Take time out – discuss with your manager about having a designated quiet area where you and other staff can go for time to yourself. You need to be clear about when this is appropriate and the procedures for letting others know where you are and how long you will be gone. Taking time out at home may be helpful too.

- Discuss your feelings with others – colleagues, friends, family (ensuring confidentiality). Your manager may be able to arrange a support group within your care setting. You should be aware of counselling services, help lines, groups, etc.

- Grieve for your losses – acknowledge grief and cry if you want to (not in front of family). Talk over grief with colleagues. Mark the person's life.

- Try to find ways to relax while away from work – this will help you to reduce stress.

- Rewarding oneself – give yourself little treats and do what you enjoy. Never feel guilty because those you care for are going through suffering and you feel you shouldn't enjoy yourself. Improving everybody's quality of life is important and that includes you.

- Be aware of your own limitations – you are not expected to know everything and cope with every situation. Know your limits and ask for support.

- Seek specialist support if signs and symptoms of stress are causing you concern.

Evidence activity

Use support systems to deal with own feelings in relation to an individual's dying or death

Explain the systems that are in place within your organisation to help you and your colleagues deal with your feelings brought on by loss and grief when providing end of life care.

Assessment summary

Your reading of this chapter and completion of the activities will have prepared you to demonstrate your learning and understanding of the principles of working in end of life care. To achieve this unit, your assessor will require you to:

Learning outcomes	Assessment criteria
Learning outcome **1**: Understand the impact of loss and grief on individuals approaching end of life by:	**1.1** describing what is meant by loss and grief before reaching end of life See Evidence activity 1.1, p.106
	1.2 explaining how the experience of loss and grief is unique to individuals and others See Evidence activity 1.2, p.106
	1.3 describing stages of loss and grief commonly experienced by individuals with a life-limiting illness See Evidence activity 1.3, p.108
	1.4 describing the effects of loss and grief on individuals and others See Evidence activity 1.4, p.109
Learning outcome **2**: Be able to support individuals through their experience of loss and grief by:	**2.1** supporting individuals and others to identify the losses they may experience See Evidence activity 2.1, p.110
	2.2 according to their preferences and wishes supporting individuals and others to communicate the losses they may experience See Evidence activity 2.2, p.111
	2.3 supporting the individual and others through each stage of grief they experience See Evidence activity 2.3, p.112
	2.4 supporting individuals and others experiencing loss and grief to access support services See Evidence activity 2.4, p.114
Learning outcome **3**: Be able to manage own feelings in relation to loss and grief by:	**3.1** describing how own feelings about loss and grief can impact on the support provided See Evidence activity 3.1, p.115
	3.2 using support systems to manage own feelings brought on by loss and grief See Evidence activity 3.2, p.116

Good luck!

Web links

Guidance for staff responsible for after death care	www.endoflifecareforadults.nhs.uk/assets/downloads/Care_After_Death___final_draft___20110610.pdf
Department of Health	www.dh.gov.uk
Macmillan Cancer Support	www.macmillan.org.uk
Marie Curie Cancer Care	www.mariecurie.org.uk
National Council for Palliative Care	www.ncpc.org.uk
National End of Life Care Programme	www.endoflifecareforadults.nhs.uk
Princess Royal Trust for Carers	www.carers.org
Dying Matters	www.dyingmatters.org
Bereavement Advice Centre	www.bereavementadvice.org
British Association for Counselling and Psychotherapy (BACP)	www.bacp.co.uk
The Compassionate Friends	www.tcf.org.uk
Cruse Bereavement Care	www.crusebereavementcare.org.uk
Institute of Family Therapy	www.instituteoffamilytherapy.org.uk
London Friend	www.londonfriend.org.uk
Samaritans	www.samaritans.org.uk
Winston's Wish	www.winstonswish.org.uk

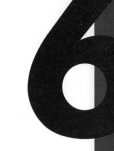

For Unit EOL 306
Support individuals during the last days of life

What are you finding out?

None of us can fully understand the feelings of someone who is dying. Most people find it difficult to know how to support someone who is facing death. It may be helpful to try to think about how you would feel if you were in that position. It is important to realise that there are no right or wrong answers to this question and every person has different priorities. This is what makes the whole subject of supporting individuals through the process of dying extremely difficult. People are unique and so are their experiences.

Caring for people towards the end of their life can be an emotional and stressful time for all concerned. Within this chapter you will explore approaches to providing care in the final hours of life and how you can support those who are left behind. You will examine the various signs that indicate a person is nearing the end of their life, as well as the comfort measures which can be taken to ensure the person experiences a good death and that the person's dignity is preserved. You will also explore the actions which must be taken following an individual's death and finally how you can manage your own feelings in relation to an individual's dying and death.

The reading and activities in this chapter will help you to:

- Understand the impact of the last days of life on the individual and others

- Understand how to respond to common symptoms in the last days of life

- Be able to support individuals and others during the last days of life

- Be able to respond to changing needs of an individual during the last days of life

- Be able to work according to national guidelines, local policies and procedures, taking into account preferences and wishes after the death of an individual

- Be able to manage your own feelings in relation to an individual's dying or death.

LO1 Understand the impact of the last days of life on the individual and others

1.1 Describe the possible psychological aspects of the dying phase for the individual and others

As the end of a person's life approaches, the person, their family and carers all need to make adjustments. Some adjustments may have already taken place over the weeks or months leading up to the dying phase; but as death approaches the reality of the situation makes things a lot more difficult for some people.

Throughout the last stage of a life-limiting illness, the person who is dying may come to realise the inevitability that death is impending and accept that it is going to happen in the very near future. During this stage, the person may express feelings of sadness and may begin to withdraw. Refusing to participate in daily activities, including personal care, is also common. The person may express a wish to be left alone.

These feelings of sadness are part of the grieving process and the person who is dying often mourns for themselves in the same way that their loved ones will grieve for their loss.

Although sadness is common, some people who believe in life after death will look forward to being reunited with loved ones who have died before them, or with their God. Some people find this belief in an afterlife comforting and reassuring.

For many people, the thought of death and dying is a frightening experience, and the nature of these fears will be unique to each individual. Some common fears about facing the end of life include fear of:

- pain
- choking or suffocation
- side effects of treatments
- losing control
- being a burden to others
- separation
- dying alone
- the unknown.

As death approaches, some people may be unable to repress painful, unresolved events, for example, a disagreement or a traumatic early life experience. The person may struggle to find peace and become restless and uneasy with the prospect of death.

Generally, most people will die as they have lived. If the person is at ease with life and has the ability to cope with stressful situations, then they will probably approach the end of their life in the same way. If, on the other hand, the person has an anxious disposition, then it is likely that the person will approach death with the same feelings. Most people approaching the end of their life will meet death with a mixture of characteristics which reflect their personality.

It is important to realise that loved ones will respond to the impending death in different ways. Some will cry, others don't; some will want to talk, others may want to remain quiet; some feel helpless and useless; some feel awkward or an urge to 'intervene'; while some will want to carry on as if everything is normal.

Loved ones may express feelings associated with guilt. They sometimes feel intense guilt about having not done more to help the person. Feelings of guilt are often more pronounced if the person facing the end of their life has had to have alternative care at the end of life. However hard the individual may have tried to look after the person at home, a feeling of failure is not uncommon at this point.

One of the most difficult emotions to deal with is that of anger. Loved ones may feel intense anger at the person who is dying for leaving them. They may be angry with the person's condition and the fact that the person is in hospital for the separation of their relationship. Equally, loved ones may express anger towards care staff for not doing enough for the individual.

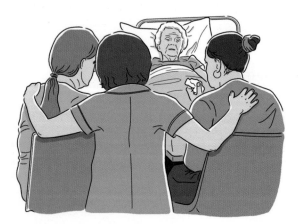

Figure 6.1 Emotional support

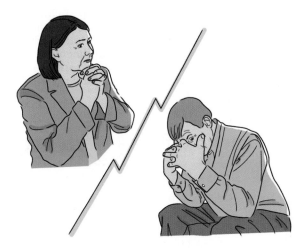

Figure 6.2 Expressions of grief

People who are facing the end of life may experience psychological reactions in relation to the impending death, the uncertainty of when the death will occur and to the physical effects of their condition.

Evidence activity

1.1 Describe the possible psychological aspects of the dying phase for the individual and others

Describe the possible emotions that a person who is facing the end of life and their loved ones might experience.

1.2 Analyse the impact of the last days of life on the relationships between individuals and others

The impact of the last few days of life on the relationship between the individual nearing the end of life and others will depend upon the nature of the individual's relationship.

The experience of living with a life-limiting illness can affect the way in which family and friends relate to each other. As the illness progresses, the life that loved ones have known together will be disrupted, as the dying person's needs become the primary focus. Roles may change as the person facing the end of life becomes more dependent upon loved ones. The illness will also affect a couple's intimacy and social life.

Watching a loved one die can be an extremely stressful experience. Depending on whom they are, who you are, and what the situation is, the stress can seem overwhelming. Not only is the person about to lose an important relationship, but they may also be forced to make major life changes. Change may not come easy. Unwanted change may be even harder to accept. And a change which threatens the person's sense of well-being is the most difficult of all.

In addition to dealing with their emotions, the individual may also be facing a host of disruptions in their daily life. The person may be responsible for extensive caregiving duties, either ones they've chosen, or ones they've inherited. Day-to-day caregiving rituals may consume the individual's thoughts and sap their energy. Financial matters may also burden them and decisions about the future may hang heavy.

Other responsibilities also vie for the individual's attention, as they may have a career to juggle, other loved ones to care for and important commitments to fulfil. Family life may be altered, if not torn apart.

What is happening to the individual nearing the end of life may cause a great deal of pain. Their disease may make them uncomfortable. Their treatments may make them sick. Their dying may make them very sad and their condition may make them unable to communicate their wishes. This may be hard to accept for individuals who are witnessing these difficult aspects, the person may no longer be recognisable and, for loved ones, changes in their relationship may be concerning. Family and friends may also distance themselves because they do not know what to say or do.

Evidence activity

1.2 Explain the impact of the last days of life on the relationships between individuals and others

How do you think the last days of a person's life might impact on their important relationships?

LO2 Understand how to respond to common symptoms in the last days of life

 Describe the common signs of approaching death

Carers and families often want to know how long their loved one 'has left', in order that they can arrange to be there and ensure other family members can be present at the time of death. An important aspect of end of life care is the notion that every person is an individual and that every person will experience death in their own unique way. There is therefore no 'standard' way of dying and attempting to assess when a person is likely to die can be very difficult, even for experienced doctors and nurses.

There are occasions when healthcare professionals have predicted that a service user will die within hours, but to their amazement the individual has continued to live for days. For some people, death may be sudden, perhaps following an acute episode such as a bleed, while for others, death will result following a long period of gradual weakening. Although this decline will be unique to each individual, there are some common signs which may indicate the person is approaching death.

Time to reflect

2.1 Signs of approaching death

Think about a time when you have provided end of life care to a person and make a note of the changes you observed, which indicated to you that the person was approaching death.

As a person approaches the very end of life, two types of signs/changes occur. There are physical changes that take place as the body begins to shut down its vital functions and there are signs/changes that take place on an emotional and spiritual level.

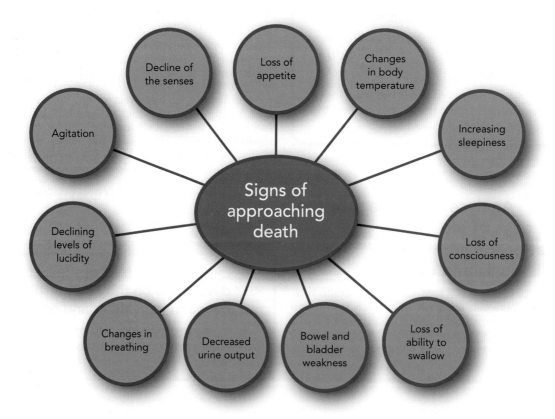

Figure 6.3 Signs of approaching death

Loss of appetite

Loss of appetite and reduced intake of food and fluid are normal as a person approaches the end of their life. As death nears, the dying person may lose interest in food and drink. The ability to swallow may also become impaired. Physically, as the body begins to shut down, the dying person may no longer want or require food and fluids. This can be a very difficult concept for carers to understand, as they become concerned that the individual will die of starvation or dehydration. At this stage, however, the body no longer needs the same level of fuel as it conserves its energy. This is nature's way of preparing for death. When a person is dying, their sensations and requirements change, so they no longer feel thirst and hunger in the way you or I would and will therefore not need to swallow fluid or food. Frequent mouth care, however, will be important at this stage in order to keep the mouth moist and alleviate any discomfort.

Changes in body temperature

As the body prepares to die, the ability to control its temperature becomes impaired, and the skin may feel clammy or cool to the touch, especially the hands, arms, legs and feet. This is a sign that the circulatory system is shutting down. At this stage, the blood is really only being circulated to the vital internal organs. The skin may also feel clammy or damp and appear blue or mottled in colour. This is usually more noticeable on the hands and feet.

Increased sleepiness and loss of consciousness

As the body begins to shut down, the individual will sleep more and communicate less. Gradually, the person will become more unresponsive as their level of consciousness decreases. Decreased movement and loss of strength can be observed and the dying person may have difficulty in responding verbally and in swallowing. It will become increasingly more difficult to wake the person and eventually the person will reach a point where they can no longer be awakened.

Loss of ability to swallow

Swallowing becomes more difficult as the person gets weaker. This can lead to the build-up of saliva and other secretions in the mouth and the back of the throat, leading to a gurgling or rattling sound with each breath the dying person takes. The noise can sound very distressing, but this is very common and is generally thought not to be uncomfortable for the dying person. Elevating and repositioning of the person's head may help to relieve some of the congestion.

Bowel and bladder weakness

As muscles weaken, the person who is dying may no longer be able to control bowel and bladder functions resulting in incontinence. This may be very distressing for the dying person and must always be handled with great care and sensitivity.

Decreased urine output

Urine output will decrease as a result of the combined effects of the kidneys beginning to fail and a decrease in fluid intake. Urine will appear dark in colour as it becomes more concentrated. Urine output may even cease entirely in the last 24 to 48 hours.

Changes in breathing

Respiration will slow down and may become laboured. The dying person's breathing pattern will also begin to change as death approaches. Breathing may become irregular, with periods of shallow and deep breaths alternating over short periods of time. During this time a person may not breathe at all for as long as 10 to 20 seconds before beginning again. This is known as Cheyne–Stokes breathing. Although 20 seconds may not sound like a long time, it is long enough that you may mistakenly think the person has died and then be startled to hear a sudden gasp and deep intake of breath. Breathing may be noisy and gurgling sounds may be heard as the dying person develops a build-up of fluid in the back of the throat and lungs. You may have heard this being referred to as the 'death rattle'. This noise can be distressing for the carers and family, but it can often be eased by changing the person's position, or treated with appropriate medication.

> ### Key terms
>
> Cheyne–Stokes breathing is an abnormal type of breathing seen especially in unconscious people, characterised by alternating periods of shallow and deep breathing.

Declining levels of perception and lucidity

As death approaches, the dying person may become disoriented. The person may not recognise his or her surroundings, become confused about time and may not even recognise family and friends. Sometimes a person who is dying may also experience hallucinations. This may take the form of talking or reaching out to something that no one else can see.

Agitation

As death approaches, some people become extremely agitated and restless. Restlessness and agitation are common and may be caused by reduced oxygen to the brain, metabolic changes, dehydration, and medication used to treat pain.

Decline of the senses

Of the five senses, vision, hearing and touch are usually those affected when a person is dying, with hearing and touch being the last two senses to deteriorate.

- **Vision** – may deteriorate slightly, and sometimes a person may experience 'visions' of people or events from the past. It is important to acknowledge what the individual is experiencing, as it will seem very real to them. Denying that the hallucinations are occurring can often be upsetting for the dying person.
- **Hearing** – of all the five senses, hearing is generally the last one to be lost. It is generally acknowledged that people who are dying can hear, even when they appear to be unconscious. It is therefore important to continue to talk to the dying person and to encourage their loved ones to do the same. However, care must be taken to ensure nothing that could upset the person is discussed.
- **Touch** – Although the dying person's arms, hands, legs and feet may feel cool, the sense of touch will still be present. A person who has slipped into unconsciousness will very often still be able to feel touch. It is therefore important to continue to gently touch the dying person, for example, by holding the person's hand, while explaining who is touching them. It is also important to encourage the dying person's loved ones to do the same.

Common signs of the last few hours of life

Common signs of the last few hours of life are as follows:

- The person is unconscious for most of the time.
- The person's urine output diminishes.
- The person's face will have a waxy appearance.
- The muscles of the person's face relax and the nose appears more prominent.
- The person's hands and feet feel cool to the touch.
- The person's breathing becomes irregular.
- The person's heart rate becomes irregular and weak.

Evidence activity

2.1 Describe the common signs of approaching death

You are required to give a talk to some new members of staff about the common signs which may indicate an individual is approaching death. Produce a hand-out which describes the common signs of approaching death to accompany your talk.

2.2 Explain how to minimise the distress of symptoms related to the last days of life

As a person nears the end of their life careful attention to symptom control is important in order to prevent, minimise or eliminate distress, thus improving quality of life up until the time of death. Because of the multidimensional nature of many symptoms, a multidisciplinary team approach to assessment and management is essential. Such a multidisciplinary team calls for the expertise of doctors, nurses, social workers, physiotherapists, dieticians and providers of spiritual care.

One of the aims of end of life care is to prevent, relieve and minimise any distress a person may be experiencing. The manifestation of distress and its causes will vary from person to person.

Distress can be physical or emotional, and can be related directly to the psychological aspects of living with a life-limiting condition or to the physical symptoms that can occur as a person is nearing the end of their life.

When a person has numerous symptoms, it is important to work with them to establish which symptom needs to be addressed first.

Distressing symptoms may include:

- pain
- weakness
- fatigue
- breathlessness
- nausea and vomiting
- skin irritations, e.g. itching

- pressure ulcers
- anorexia (loss of appetite)
- mouth problems (ulcers and sores).

When caring for service users who are experiencing distressing symptoms, it is important first to determine the cause of the symptom. If a person is experiencing pain, it is likely that they will be prescribed medication and, in some instances, very strong analgesics.

A side effect of these types of medication is constipation. This could lead to further distress as the person becomes impacted by faeces.

If the cause of the symptom is known, steps can be taken to alleviate the distress. Often it is the not knowing what the problem is that can cause more distress than the symptom itself. Not all symptoms can be alleviated with medication.

Some symptoms can be relieved by simple measures such as repositioning the person for comfort and to prevent the formation of pressure ulcers. Equally, moistening the person's mouth and lips can help to prevent and alleviate a sore mouth.

In order to fully support a person with symptoms that may cause distress, it is crucial that they are observed in order that changes in their needs are recognised at an early stage. Some symptoms may get worse, and new symptoms may also appear.

It is therefore essential that health and social care workers fully observe individuals in order that appropriate support can be offered as soon as possible, thus minimising the extent of any distress caused.

Evidence activity

 Explain how to minimise the distress of symptoms related to the last days of life

Think about a service user who is receiving end of life care. Identify any distressing symptoms you have observed them experiencing. Explain how you have supported the person to alleviate their symptoms and any associated distress.

- What were the symptoms?
- What measures did you take?
- How effective were the measures?
- Did you need to involve any other services, for example, physiotherapist, doctor, palliative care nurse?

2.3 ## Describe appropriate comfort measures in the final hours of life

During the final hours of their life, most people will require continuous skilled care. This care can be delivered in any setting, provided care professionals, the family and carers are appropriately prepared and supported throughout the process. An essential part of this care involves measures to ensure the comfort of the person who is dying. The goal of ensuring comfort measures is to focus on keeping the dying person as comfortable as possible, prevent or relieve suffering as much as possible, while respecting the dying person's wishes. Thus ensuring everything is done to ensure the person experiences a 'good death'.

Discomfort can occur for a variety of reasons, for example, pain, nausea, fatigue, difficulty with swallowing, eating and drinking, constipation and incontinence. Recognising the causes of discomfort and applying appropriate comfort measures can help to relieve unnecessary suffering.

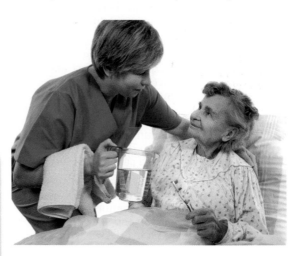

Figure 6.4 Comfort measures

The challenge to members of the care team is to continually review the person who is dying and critically observe any changes in their condition, in order that appropriate comfort measures can be instigated as soon as possible.

Some of the causes of discomfort and the comfort measures which can be undertaken are given in Table 6.1.

Table 6.1 Causes of discomfort at the end of life and suggested comfort measures

Aspect of care	Suggested comfort measures
Pain relief	Pain is subjective and is very real to the individual person. Pain should be assessed on a regular basis, in order to establish the location, cause, type and severity of the pain. Pain medication is required until death. It is always better to administer medication in anticipation of the pain, rather than waiting for pain to occur. If pain is not well controlled, this must be reported to the individual's doctor in order that the pain control can be reviewed. In the last days, the person may not be able to swallow pain medication. When service users cannot take medicines by mouth, the pain medication may be given by other routes, for example, by placing it under the tongue or into the rectum, by injection or infusion, or by placing a patch on the skin.
Food and fluid intake	It is important to resist the urge to force the person to eat or drink. Going without food and water is generally not painful, and eating can add to discomfort. Loss of appetite is a common and natural part of dying. Offer only what the person wants.
Dysphagia (difficulty swallowing)	Offer only what the person can handle. If the person has lost the ability to swallow it is essential that food and fluids are not given by mouth, as this will most definitely lead to choking. A person who experiences difficulty with swallowing must be assessed by a speech and language therapist, who will be able to give advice on techniques for feeding and the types and textures of food and fluids that can be safely given. As dehydration is inevitable, it is important to ensure the mouth and lips are kept moist. You should therefore moisten the mouth with a swab and lubricate the lips with lip balm.
Mouth care	Medication, treatment, disease symptoms, breathing through an open mouth, or a combination of all of these problems, can lead to a dry mouth. Unattended it will lead to discomfort and discourage a good dietary intake. A dry mouth will also increase the risk of mouth ulcers and thrush developing. Regular cleaning of the mouth is important. This should include brushing teeth and tongue and using a mouth rinse. Dentures should be removed and thoroughly cleaned. Vaseline or flavoured lip balm should be used to keep the lips moist. Sucking small pieces of ice can help to keep the mouth moist. If the person is semi-conscious, confused or asleep do not put fluids into the mouth, as the person may inhale the fluid. The mouth can be kept moist with a dampened oral sponge or swab.
Breathing	If the person has developed a rattle when breathing it may help to turn the person on their side to allow the saliva to drain from the mouth. If this does not help, communicate with the person's doctor in order that medication that will dry up the secretions can be prescribed. Explain to the family that due to the person's decreased level of consciousness this is not distressing for the person who is dying. If the person is experiencing breathlessness, opening a window or using a fan to increase air circulation can help. A calm, uncluttered environment can help the person experiencing breathlessness. Avoid asking questions which require a lengthy answer. Where possible, avoid or assist with activities which make breathlessness worse. Always ensure the person can reach a call bell when you are not in the room.
Elimination	A person who is approaching the end of their life may lose control of their bowel and bladder function. Equally, urine output may decrease and become dark in colour. The person may also experience constipation. Incontinence can be very distressing to the person and can also increase risks associated with the development of pressure ulcers. It is important that appropriate continence aids are used to ensure comfort. Unless an advance decision has been made by the dying person regarding catheterisation, a decision may be made to insert a urinary catheter.

Aspect of care	Suggested comfort measures
Skin care	The use of pressure-relieving aids can assist in the prevention of pressure ulcers. As death approaches, the person should be assisted to reposition for comfort only, supporting with pillows where appropriate. Ensure pressure areas are cushioned. Skin should be kept clean and special attention should be paid to creases and folds in the skin. It is essential that a good skin-care routine is observed in order to prevent the development of pressure ulcers or breaks in the skin.
Increased levels of sleep	It is important to continue to talk to the person, as it is possible that they are still able to hear you even if they appear to be asleep. Encourage the family to do the same. Short conversations can be planned for times when the person is more alert.
Confusion, disorientation and agitation	Some causes are reversible, for example, a urinary tract infection can lead to confusion. Reversible causes should always be investigated and treated. If there are no reversible causes, sedation may be helpful in settling the person. Be aware of your care approach and the effect this can have on the person. Give plenty of reassurance and be mindful of the wishes of the person as to the things they want or need prior to death. Ensure the environment remains calm as a bustling and stressful environment can make things worse for the person.

Evidence activity

 Describe appropriate comfort measures in the final hours of life

Take a look at the following aspects of care and suggest one comfort measure that you could offer as a person enters the final days or hours of their life.

Aspect of care	Suggested comfort measures
Pain relief	
Food and fluid intake	
Dysphagia (difficulty swallowing)	
Mouth care	
Breathing	
Elimination	
Skin care	
Increased levels of sleep	
Confusion, disorientation and agitation	

2.4 **Explain the circumstances when life-prolonging treatment can be stopped or withheld**

As an individual nears the end of their life, there will be times when difficult decisions need to be made in relation to stopping or withholding treatment.

Life-prolonging treatment can be stopped or withheld:

- **When a person refuses to accept treatment** – a person who is deemed competent to make decisions has the right to refuse treatment.

- **When a person does not have capacity but has made an advance decision to refuse treatment** – as long as a valid advance decision to refuse treatment was completed when the person had capacity, the healthcare team are legally obliged to conform to these decisions.

- **When medical intervention is of no overall benefit to the person** – it is the duty of the doctor in charge of the individual's care to recognise when treatment should be withheld or withdrawn. There may be times when treatment may prolong life; however, the quality of life may be so poor that the person may live their remaining time in severe pain or perhaps in a semi-conscious state. In this type of situation, the treatment has no overall benefit to the person and it may be decided in the best interest of the person that certain treatments should be stopped or withheld. These decisions are never taken lightly and always involve careful consultation.

Evidence activity

2.4 Explain the circumstances when life-prolonging treatment can be stopped or withheld

Explain three circumstances under which life-prolonging treatment can be stopped or withheld.

 2.5 **Identify the signs that death has occurred**

The moment of death can be a very emotional as well as confusing moment for health and social care workers. Many comment that they feel lost for words, often not knowing what to say or how to react. Some deaths happen suddenly and some

are distressing until the end. However, most people slip into a state of unawareness. The following are all signs that death has occurred.

- The person will be unresponsive.
- There will be no pulse.
- The person will not be breathing.
- The person's eyes will be fixed and may be open or closed.
- The person's jaw will become slack.
- There may be a loss of control of the bladder and bowel.
- The person will feel cool as the body temperature drops.
- The person's skin colour will change as the blood settles, the person's skin will be paler, bluish and then a whitish or ashen grey.

Evidence activity

2.5 Identify the signs that death has occurred

You are supporting a service user who is nearing the end of life. What signs would you look for to establish whether the person has died?

LO3 Be able to support individuals and others during the last days of life

 3.1 **Demonstrate a range of ways to enhance an individual's well-being during the last days of life**

Emotional well-being refers to a sense of balance in a person's life; between solitude and sociability, work and play, sleep and wakefulness, rest and exercise. It is about how we feel, think and behave, particularly when faced with life's challenges and adversities. A person in good emotional health is more likely to engage in productive activities, have fulfilling relationships, feel good about themselves and care for themselves and others.

When our emotional or psychological well-being is compromised this can have detrimental effects on the individual's sense of worth and can further compound the person's physical health.

Environmental factors

The environment can have an enormous impact on a person's well-being as they approach the end of their life. An environment which promotes inclusion and participation will enable the individual to remain an active partner in planning care. An environment which is clinical and cold is likely to reinforce to the person that they are living with an illness, while an environment which is homely and warm is more likely to enhance the person's well-being. For some people, it may be particularly important that they can get outside. A sensory garden can provide the senses with different colours, smells, sounds and textures. Ensuring the environment is calm and relaxed can also help to reduce feelings of anxiety. Soft music and aromatherapy can be very soothing for some people.

Non-medical interventions

Non-medical interventions can be used to enhance an individual's well-being, but will depend on the individual and their abilities. For some people, just having someone there for them can have an enormous impact on their sense of well-being. For someone to hold the person's hand, if this is acceptable to the person, can also be soothing. There are many ways in which symptoms can be relieved using non-medical interventions; for example, a person who is experiencing difficulty with breathing can be supported to reposition so the person is sitting upright, which can alleviate the distress that comes with being breathless.

For some individuals, prayer can be extremely comforting, and a visit from the individual's religious representative may help them to feel positive and more relaxed.

Equipment and aids

The use of equipment and aids can help a person to maintain their independence; for example, assistive technology can be used to remind a person it is the right time to take their medication. Without certain pieces of equipment, some service users may require the assistance of health and social care staff, which could take away their independence. A person who is experiencing breathlessness may benefit from the use of a nebuliser or equally an electric fan may help to reduce the feelings of anxiety associated with shortness of breath.

Alternative therapies

Alternative therapies are also referred to as unconventional therapies. These therapies are used instead of conventional treatments. There are many reasons why people choose alternative therapies. Some people are afraid of conventional treatments for fear of side effects. Alternative therapies can enhance a person's sense of well-being because they very often focus on the whole person and not just the treatment of the condition.

Evidence activity

3.1 Give examples of how an individual's well-being can be enhanced

This activity will help you to demonstrate your knowledge of factors which can enhance an individual's well-being.

Think about your service users and, in particular, a person who is nearing the end of their life. Give examples of factors which can enhance the life of individuals, taking into account:

- the environment
- non-medical interventions
- equipment and aids
- alternative therapies.

3.2 Work in partnership with others to support the individual's well-being

The provision of good end of life care requires a team approach and should incorporate the expertise and skills from a number of different disciplines. In addition to drawing upon the skills of doctors, nurses and carers, good end of life care will also require the skills of other professionals such as physiotherapists, complementary therapists, chaplaincy services and professional counselling services. Central to achieving this aim is ensuring effective co-ordination of care across all teams and providers who are involved in the care of service users and their family.

Partnership working is an essential aspect in supporting people who are nearing the end of their life. The partners that you work with may include:

- the individuals you support, their carers, family and friends
- your colleagues and other members of the immediate care team
- members of the specialist palliative care team

- hospital staff
- the individual's GP
- advocacy services.

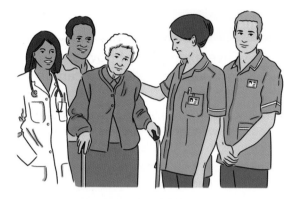

Figure 6.5 Partnership working

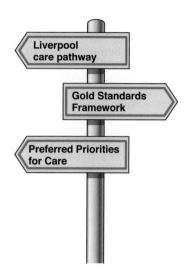

Figure 6.6 End of life care tools

The most important people in partnership working are the individuals you support and the people who are important to them. If these people feel they are actively participating in the partnership, this can have a dramatic effect on their overall health and well-being.

Evidence activity

 3.2 **Work in partnership with others to support the individual's well-being**

Make a note of how you work in partnership with key people to support the well-being of individuals receiving end of life care.

3.3 **Describe how to use a range of tools for end of life care according to agreed ways of working**

Three of the most well-known tools are the:
- Gold Standards Framework (GSF)
- Liverpool Care Pathway (LCP)
- Preferred Priorities for Care document.

The Gold Standards Framework

The Gold Standards Framework was initially developed for use in primary care settings so that people approaching the end of life could be identified and their care needs assessed, in order that a plan of care could be drawn up and appropriate agencies put into place. The principles of the Gold Standards Framework have been adapted for various settings and can be used in primary care, care homes, acute hospitals, prisons and for all individuals regardless of their diagnosis.

The overall aims of the Gold Standard Framework are to:
- improve the quality of care for individuals who are nearing the end of their lives
- improve coordination and collaboration with all members of the care team
- reduce the number of people who are unnecessarily transferred to hospital in the last stages of life.

The Gold Standards Framework involves three steps that are facilitated by effective and clear communication. It aims to:
1. Identify people in need of end of life care.
2. Assess and record the needs and preferences of the individual.
3. Plan and provide care appropriate to the individual's needs.

The five goals of the Gold Standard Framework aim to ensure:

1. The service user's symptoms are controlled.
2. The service user is enabled to choose their preferred priorities for care and where they would like to spend the last phase of their life.
3. The service user feels safe and secure, with fewer episodes of crisis.
4. The carers feel supported, involved, empowered and satisfied.
5. There is enhanced confidence and teamwork among the carers and communication and collaboration with other professionals are maximised.

In order to achieve these objectives, the Gold Standard Framework has established seven core standards; also known as the seven Cs. These are shown in Table 6.2.

The Liverpool Care Pathway

The Liverpool Care Pathway was established by a specialist palliative care team at the Royal Liverpool and Broadgreen University Hospitals and the team at the Liverpool Marie Curie Centre. The aim of the team was to develop a pathway that health professionals could follow in the last days or hours of a person's life. The Liverpool Care Pathway is therefore a tool that can be used

Table 6.2 Core standards of the Gold Standard Framework

The seven core standards of the Gold Standard Framework are:	
C1: Communication	Care settings using the Gold Standards Framework maintain a Supportive Care Register to record, plan and evaluate the care of people who are receiving end of life care. The register is also used to facilitate discussions surrounding the person's care within regular team meetings.
C2: Coordination	Each team should have a nominated person to coordinate and oversee the organisation and smooth running of the framework.
C3: Control of symptoms	Every person requiring end of life care should have their symptoms and any associated problems assessed, recorded, discussed and acted upon in accordance with the agreed strategy. The control of symptoms should take into account emotional, social, psychological and spiritual needs as well as physical.
C4: Continuity of care	Continuity of care includes out-of-hours care and staff should be aware of what help is available out of hours and how speedily this can be accessed. This is important in helping to prevent unnecessary admissions to hospital. The person and immediate family should be provided with a pack, which details important telephone numbers and a 'who's who', in addition to what to do and who to contact in an emergency.
C5: Continued learning	In order to provide a high standard of end of life care, staff must be given the opportunity to access resources to keep their knowledge and skills up to date. Staff must also be given the opportunity to discuss, learn from and reflect on their experiences, in order to identify areas of best practice and also to identify areas for further development.
C6: Carer support	Supporting carers is an essential part of end of life care. Practical and emotional support should be made available to carers throughout the process of caring and also in the form of bereavement care following the death of their loved one.
C7: Care in the dying phase	C7 is a natural extension of the other six core standards. Every person entering the final days of life must be appropriately cared for. This is the time when non-essential drug interventions are discontinued. Care focuses on ensuring the person is as comfortable as possible and ensuring spiritual and emotional needs are being met. The Gold Standards Framework recommends the implementation of the Liverpool Care Pathway at this point.

for all people who are in their last days of life, irrespective of their primary disease or the cause of their imminent death.

The Liverpool Care Pathway for the Dying Person was developed to transfer the hospice model of care into other care settings. It is recognised nationally and internationally as leading practice in care of the dying to enable people to die a dignified death and provide support to their relatives and carers.

The Liverpool Care Pathway provides guidance on the different aspects of care, including:

- comfort measures
- symptom control
- anticipatory prescribing of medication and the discontinuation of inappropriate interventions
- emotional and spiritual support
- communication with the dying person and their loved ones
- communication with the Primary Health Care Team.

Preferred Priorities for Care

The 'Preferred Priorities for Care' is a person-held document and was designed to facilitate choice in relation to end of life care. It can help individuals who are living with a life-limiting illness to prepare for their future. It gives them an opportunity to think about, talk about and write down their preferences and priorities for care at the end of their life.

The Preferred Priorities for Care can help carers to understand what is important to the individual when planning care. If a time comes when, for whatever reason, the individual is unable to make a decision for themselves, anyone who has to make decisions about care on the individual's behalf will have to take into account anything the person has written in their Preferred Priorities for Care. The document is updated as required and travels with the individual throughout their pathway of care.

Evidence activity

3.3 Describe how to use a range of tools for end of life care according to agreed ways of working

Think about the end of life care tools used within your workplace and describe how these tools are used according to agreed ways of working.

3.4 Support others to understand the process following death according to agreed ways of working

Following the death of a person, there are many arrangements and decisions to be made, all of which can be extremely difficult in a time of grief.

Following the death of their loved one, relatives will eventually return home, and it is important that they have clear instructions which detail what they need to do next. Because people who are distressed have difficulty retaining verbal information, it is really helpful if you can give them written information on when they can collect the death certificate and how and where to register the death. The following information would be helpful to a person who is newly bereaved.

It is highly unlikely that you are going to be involved personally in registering a person's death. In fact, deaths are most commonly registered by a relative of the deceased. However, it is important to have a general awareness of the procedure, as this will help you to answer any questions that may be asked by bereaved relatives within your workplace.

When a person has died, the doctor who has attended the individual during their illness will issue a death certificate. However, this can only be issued provided the cause of death is natural and the deceased has been seen by the doctor in the 14 days prior to death.

If the individual died in the community, the person's GP will issue the death certificate. If the death took place in hospital, depending on the time, the death certificate may not be issued immediately and bereaved relatives may need to return the following day to collect the certificate. Most hospitals will have an office from which the certificate can be collected.

Registering a death in England and Wales

Once the death certificate has been issued the death must then be registered with the Registrar of Births, Deaths and Marriages in the sub-district in which the death occurred. The death must be registered within five days and is usually registered by a relative of the deceased, unless the death has been referred to a coroner. If there are no relatives then it is possible for another individual to register the death, for example, someone who was present at the death.

In order that the death can be registered the Registrar will want to know:

- the date and place of death
- the name and address of the deceased (if the deceased was a married female her maiden name will also need to be disclosed)
- the deceased's date and place of birth
- the deceased person's occupation or last known occupation
- details of any state pension or allowance from public funds
- the date of birth of any surviving spouse
- the deceased person's marital status
- if the deceased was a woman, the occupation of her husband.

In addition, the Registrar will also want to see:

- the death certificate issued by the doctor
- the person's medical card, birth certificate, marriage certificate if available, and war pension order book if the person had one
- the Form 100 issued by the coroner, if the death had been referred to a coroner.

After completing the registration, the Registrar will issue:

- A certificate for burial or cremation, known as the 'green form', giving permission for the body to be buried or to apply for the body to be cremated. This certificate is free, but if additional copies are requested these will be provided for a fee.
- A certificate of registration of death, which is used for social security purposes if the person was on a state pension or benefits.

Registering a death in Scotland

In Scotland the death must be registered within eight days. The information required by the Registrar is much the same as in England and Wales; however, some additional information is also required. This includes information relating to the time of death and other family members. Following registration the Registrar will issue a Certificate of Registration of Death, which is given to the funeral director. The Registrar will also issue a Registration or Notification of Death form, which is used for obtaining or adjusting benefits, or for National Insurance purposes.

Registering a death in Northern Ireland

The procedures for registering a death in Northern Ireland are very similar to those in England and Wales. The death must be registered within five days. However, doctors can provide a Medical Death Certificate if they have attended the person in the 28 days before their death.

Evidence activity

 3.4 Support others to understand the process following death according to agreed ways of working

Explain how individuals are supported through the processes that follow death within your place of work.

LO4 Be able to respond to changing needs of an individual during the last days of life

4.1 Explain the importance of following the individual's advance care plan in the last days of life

Broadly speaking, the aim of end of life care is to ensure that a person's whole care needs are met in a holistic manner, and that the person has the choice to be cared for and die where they wish and as they would wish.

An advance care plan will detail the individual's wishes about his or her future health care and would have been written in consultation with the health care team, family members and other important people in their lives. The advance care plan offers the individual the opportunity to say now what life-prolonging medical treatment they would and would not want in the future. If in the future the individual is unable to express their wishes about treatment, their doctor and family will know what they would have wanted or how they would have liked the choices to be made.

The individual may have expressed wishes and preferences in relation to future treatment and care, who they want to be involved in future decision making, types of treatment they may or may not wish to receive and where the individual wishes to receive care.

Having these decisions in writing can make the individual's wishes clear to both the family and the health care team. It can also lower the levels of stress for both the individual and the family.

In the last days of life an individual may be unable to make decisions or make their wishes and preferences known due to loss of consciousness, and it is at this point that health care staff will rely on the advance care plan to ensure the individual's wishes and preferences are implemented. It is therefore of utmost importance that the individual's preferences and wishes are respected in order to ensure appropriate care needs are supported and to avoid unnecessary distress by administering treatments that the individual would not have wanted. Advance care planning is an important tool in enabling the individual to remain autonomous at a time when their ability to make decisions and to give consent is compromised.

Evidence activity

 4.1 Explain the importance of following the individual's advance care plan in the last days of life

Why do you think it is important that an individual's advance care plan is followed in the last days of life?

 4.2 Record the changing needs of the individual according to agreed ways of working

Every person within your workplace will have a care plan or a support plan. This describes the service user's needs and how they should be met. The care plan tells anyone involved with the care of the service user about the level of support that must be given. Care plans cover every aspect of a service user's life. The purpose of a care plan is to provide a detailed written record of the individual's needs and wishes and identify the level of support that a person requires with their health, personal and social care needs.

Among other things, care plans cover:

- mobility
- continence
- washing and dressing
- social activities
- communication
- medication
- spiritual needs
- religious and cultural needs
- health.

Everyone who is involved in the individual's care is likely to want to look at their care plan, in order to ensure that they are providing the right support and following the individual's wishes. Depending on the person's needs, several people may look at the care plan, such as the GP, palliative care nurse, speech therapist, dietician, physiotherapist and occupational therapist.

In many organisations the individual's care plan is updated daily by care or nursing staff. In this case the care plan will include blank forms, which can be filled in to show the support the person has received that day and any changes in the service user's condition.

The information that is recorded daily will be used to make appropriate changes to the care plan when it is reviewed. Therefore, it is essential that the information you record about the changing needs of the individual is:

- legible, so that everyone can read what has been written
- accurate and factual
- complete, with all the necessary facts but without unnecessary waffle
- signed and dated, so that others can check with you if they have any questions about the information.

Case Study

4.2 Mrs Riaz

Today you have assisted Mrs Riaz with her personal care needs. While you were assisting her, you noticed that she appears more withdrawn than usual. She is not interested in going to the bathroom but does agree to have a wash in bed. She normally sits out in her chair but has expressed a wish to remain in bed today. This is not a usual occurrence, so you reported it to your manager. The manager has asked you to record the information in Mrs Riaz' care plan.

Write down what you would record in the care plan and why.

Evidence activity

 4.2 **Record the changing needs of the individual according to agreed ways of working**

Explain the requirements for recording the changing needs of individuals within your workplace.

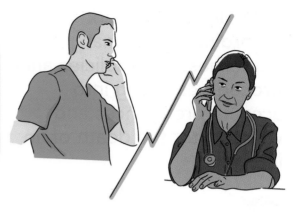

Figure 6.7 Reporting changes

4.3 Support the individual when their condition changes according to agreed ways of working

In the final stages of many life-limiting conditions, care priorities tend to shift. Instead of ongoing curative measures, the focus often changes to palliative care for the relief of pain symptoms, and emotional stress. It is important that staff deal with these as they arise.

As a person nears the end of their life their condition may change at differing rates and with different levels of severity. Many physical changes occur during the process of dying that affect the emotional, social, and spiritual aspects of a person's life. It is therefore important to know when to take appropriate action when a person's condition changes.

Using your skills to critically observe the person will help you to detect changes as they occur.

Any changes must then be reported to the appropriate person, in order to ensure the person's end of life care needs continue to be coordinated and met. This may include changes in physical condition, which may require the input of a doctor, for example, if pain is not very well controlled; or the individual may require further assessment following deterioration in their mobility. This may also extend to informing relatives if the individual's condition has changed so much that they need to come into the care facility, in order to guarantee they can be present at the time of death.

It is also essential that any changes in the individual's condition are recorded within their care plan or support plan, in order to ensure the changes are communicated to other members of the care team.

It is important to realise that the provision of care must be delivered by multiple disciplines, all of which will bring their own skills and qualities. End of life care cannot be provided by one person alone.

Evidence activity

4.3 **Take appropriate action when a patient's condition changes, according to agreed ways of working**

Think about a person for whom you have been involved in their end of life care. In particular, think about a time when their condition changed. What actions were taken at that point?

LO5 Be able to work according to national guidelines, local policies and procedures taking into account preferences and wishes after the death of an individual

 Implement actions immediately after a death that respect the individual's wishes according to agreed ways of working

Many people have had no experience of being there when someone dies, or having to deal with the practical aspects that follow death. They can become extremely worried that they do not follow the correct procedures and this can be in addition to having mixed emotions about the death of the individual.

Your workplace will have its own policies and procedures relating to what to do immediately following a person's death. Once a person's death has occurred, there are a number of steps that need to be followed.

- If you work in a care home or the community, the most senior member of staff should contact the deceased person's GP, who will certify the death. It is important to explain that a death has occurred and that a doctor is required to visit as soon as possible. If the death occurs out of surgery hours, there should be a recorded message, which will provide the details of who to contact out of hours.
- The time of death and the people present must be recorded in the individual's care notes.
- If not present, the next of kin must be contacted.
- Care after death must be performed according to the individual's personal beliefs, religious beliefs and any special requirements.

- Ensure that any personal belongings are collected and recorded and are carefully packaged ready to give to relatives.
- Ensure that relatives are fully supported in any way they need, for example, you may be asked to provide information regarding registering the death and funeral arrangements.

Research and investigate

 The main points of your organisation's policy for performing care after death

Refer to your organisation's policy for performing care after death. What are the main points of this policy?

Evidence activity

Describe the steps that need to be taken immediately after a death has occurred

Describe the steps you should take following the death of a service user.

Research and investigate

 Respecting religious and cultural beliefs

Using any resources available to you, make a poster to indicate the after-death care requirements of the following religions:

- Christianity
- Buddhism
- Hinduism
- Sikhism
- Islamism
- Judaism

5.2 Provide care for the individual after death according to national guidelines, local policies and procedures

When a person dies all staff need to follow good practice, which includes being responsive to the individual's wishes for their after-death care. In relation to the individual, care after death includes:

- honouring the spiritual or cultural wishes of the deceased person
- preparing the body for transfer to the mortuary, or the funeral director's premises
- offering family and carers present the opportunity to participate in the process and supporting them to do so
- ensuring that the privacy and dignity of the deceased person is maintained
- ensuring that the health and safety of everyone who comes into contact with the body is protected
- honouring people's wishes for organ and tissue donation
- returning the deceased person's personal possessions to their relatives.

National guidance for staff responsible for care after death is available from the National End of Life Care Programme. This guidance reinforces the fact that the end of life is not when care stops. The care provided after death is also important. Members of staff with responsibility for care after death need to understand how the body should be prepared before being transferred, as well as other activities which also need to be carried out in a sensitive manner. Procedures for care after death should also be set out in thorough policies within your organisation.

Remember, the way in which you treat the deceased will not only demonstrate the respect you have for the person's wishes, but will also have an impact on the grieving process for the bereaved.

Evidence activity

 5.2 Provide care for the individual after death according to national guidelines, local policies and procedures

Explain how after-death care is provided according to national guidelines and local policies and procedures within your organisation.

5.3 Explain the importance of following the advance care plan to implement the individual's preferences and wishes for their after death care

Good end of life care does not stop at the point of death. When a person dies, it is important that all caregivers provide the highest standard of care and follow good practice. This includes ensuring the preferences and wishes of the individual are considered throughout their after death care.

After death care extends beyond the physical aspects of preparing the body for transfer to the mortuary or the funeral directors. It is therefore important that any spiritual, cultural or practical wishes the dying person and their family may have are identified and documented prior to death. This is usually undertaken as part of the advance care planning process and may include issues such as urgent release for burial or cremation, or specific wishes regarding organ donation, tissue and body donation and post mortem examination.

It is therefore essential that members of staff are aware of the advance care plan and the wishes of the individual in order that specific preferences and wishes as this will influence the way in which carers meet the needs of the individual as death approaches and afterwards. It will also ensure that members of staff are able to meet the bereavement needs of the individual's family and ensure the individual's experience of death is a good one.

Evidence activity

 5.3 Explain the importance of following the advance care plan to implement the individual's preferences and wishes for their after death care

Explain why following the after death care according to the individual's wishes and preferences and in accordance with their advance care plan is important.

5.4 Follow any agreed ways of working relating to prevention and control of infection when caring for and transferring a deceased person

Your workplace should have a policy relating to infection prevention and control and it is essential that you refer to and follow this policy when caring for and transferring the body of a person who has died.

As well as ensuring the care given to the deceased person focuses on their cultural and religious beliefs, you also have a responsibility to ensure you fulfil health and safety requirements.

All staff who are responsible for caring for and transferring a deceased person must practise standard infection control precautions. This includes treating every person as if they are potentially infectious and taking appropriate precautions to minimise the spread of micro-organisms. In order to practise standard infection control precautions, you must make appropriate use of personal protective equipment, that is, disposable gloves and apron. If there is a risk of splashing, then protective eyewear must be worn.

The standard hygienic preparation of a body usually involves the washing of the deceased, closing eyes and mouth, tidying the hair and possibly shaving the face. In the case of cultural and religious ritual some significant others may want to prepare the body before burial.

There is a need to maintain the confidentiality of a patient's medical condition, even after their death. At the same time, there is obligation to inform personnel who may be at risk of infection through contact with dead bodies so that appropriate measures may be taken to guard against infection. If family members wish to prepare the body, you must ensure that they are aware of the risks and that appropriate Infection Control Precautions are followed.

Most bodies are not infectious; however, through the natural process of decomposition the body may become a source of potential infection, whether previously infected or not; also not all cases of infection may have been identified before death; therefore, standard precautions should be used routinely.

Micro-organisms in or on a deceased person's body are unlikely to infect healthy people with intact skin, but there are other ways they may be spread, for example, through:

- needle-stick injuries with a contaminated instrument or sharp fragment of bone
- intestinal pathogens from anal and oral orifices
- abrasions, wounds and sores on the skin
- splashes or aerosols onto the eyes.

In order to prevent risks associated with the spread of micro-organisms, it is therefore important that you:

- Adopt the same standard routine protective precautions as when the individual was alive – including CE-marked disposable gloves and a disposable plastic apron when handling the deceased. Any surface contamination should be removed by washing.
- Cover any wounds or leaking openings with occlusive dressings.
- Take care to avoid contamination of any wounds or skin lesions on your hands.
- Thoroughly wash your hands following handling the deceased person's body.
- Remove all drains, catheters and intravenous lines if the death has not been reported to the Coroner.

There may be times when the body will need to be placed in a body bag prior to transferring to the mortuary. Plastic body bags are used for bodies which are known or thought to be infective to handlers, likely to leak in transit and should only be used for cases where a risk assessment makes it necessary. Body bags which are used inappropriately for bodies that are of minimal, or no, risk may cause problems to mortuary staff and may cause distress to relatives. Bodies cool more slowly inside a body bag, facilitating decomposition and making hygienic preparation more difficult. It may only be possible to display the head for viewing and this may cause additional distress to the bereaved.

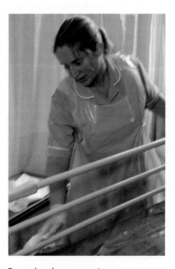

Figure 6.8 Standard precautions

If a person has died with a known or suspected infection, it is essential and a legal responsibility that all persons who may be involved in handling the body are informed of the potential risk of infection. They should be advised of the risks of infection, but the specific diagnosis remains confidential, even after death.

■ Research and investigate

5.4 Find out about the correct procedure for the use, removal and disposal of PPE

What is the correct procedure for the use, removal and disposal of PPE within your organisation?

Evidence activity

5.4 Follow any agreed ways of working relating to prevention and control of infection when caring for and transferring a deceased person

Take a look at your organisation's policy relating to infection prevention and control when caring for and transferring the body of a deceased person and make a note of the standard precautions that you need to take, in order to minimise risks to yourself and others required to handle the body.

5.5 **Explain ways to support others immediately following the death of the individual**

■ Research and investigate

5.5 Providing support

Locate your organisation's policy for supporting family and friends following the death of a service user. What are the key points of this policy?

When death occurs, the person's muscles will relax, breathing will stop, the heart will stop beating, and there will be no pulse. Even when death is expected, shock and disbelief is still common. Hospice staff or the person's doctor should be notified within a few hours, but a natural death is certainly not an emergency and the medical team do not need to be called immediately. Many people find it comforting to take some time to sit with their loved one, perhaps talking quietly, just holding hands, or seeing their loved one at peace.

The period immediately following a person's death can be a very emotional time for all involved, including family, friends, other service users and care staff. This is perfectly understandable and it is not unusual for care workers to feel as though they do not know what to say to families. There are many ways in which you can help ease the distress of family and friends.

Some relatives may choose to visit for shorter periods and go home at night, so may not be present if the individual dies overnight. Every single person has his or her own way of coping with the situation. Relatives may express a wish to be contacted at the time of death. It is therefore very important that an accurate record be kept in the individual's notes. This should include:

- next of kin details
- telephone number and address details of persons to be contacted.

It is vital that you know who you should contact first if the individual's condition deteriorates. Relatives should also be asked whether they would like to be called out during the night, and their wishes should all be documented clearly and accurately within the individual's notes. It is vital to know who to notify in the event of deterioration of a person's general condition, or that individual's death and when it is acceptable to make contact, that is, time of the day or night. Telephoning the wrong person at an inappropriate time (e.g. a frail, elderly wife/husband at 3.00 am) may cause distress. Loved ones who wished to be notified of a person's death, or wanted to be present as the individual passes away, regardless of the time of day or night may be very upset if they are not notified.

Do not assume that relatives will notify each other. Always check that the family member contacted will take responsibility for informing other family members. If relatives are present at the time of death, always ask if they wish to use the telephone, or if there is anyone they would like you to contact. This is particularly important if a relative or friend is there alone. It is essential that you remain calm and show compassion and empathy.

Family and friends may want to spend time with the individual at the time of death and afterwards. They should be fully supported to do this if they wish. It is important to ensure a key staff member is available and prepared for different responses to the death.

Offer refreshments and provide a quiet space. Any conversations or meetings with relatives should be free from interruption. Ensure that they are given clear information and the person knows what to do next and where they need to go. Answer any questions and check the person has understood. It is vital to make sure that information is given at the appropriate moment. Give the person time to collect their thoughts, talk about their feelings and deal with their distress before you ask sensitive questions and give information. Listen, and let them talk about their relatives and their feelings. Ask for the support of senior colleagues whenever you need it.

Never expect all people to react in the same way; some may not wish to sit with the person as they die or stay with the deceased. The important thing is that the person is not left to die alone, and that any relatives are comforted if they choose not to stay in the room as death approaches and afterwards.

Relatives should know where to collect the death certificate (if this is not available to give to them at the time), where and how to register the death. Straightforward, written instructions may be helpful and will give information that a distressed relative may have forgotten. Your manager will advise relatives and you can help by passing on any concerns or questions loved ones may have.

The deceased's property should be packed tidily and a list made. Your organisation should have a policy on the return of property, including flowers, food, confectionery and drinks. If these are not returned and not requested, keep them in case they are required in the following few days. The use of black bin bags is not allowed. Rinse through any soiled clothing and put in a sealed bag; mention this to relatives, as they may not wish to have such items returned to them – however, do not assume this.

Check that people are not leaving alone or driving if they are distressed. Wherever possible, it should be arranged for someone to accompany them, pick them up or meet them at home. However, if a person insists they wish to be alone respect this. Report to your manager and keep them informed at all times; they will be able to advise and assist relatives. Your manager may phone the person later to see if they arrived safely and need anything and/or anyone.

Case Study

 Shamus

Shamus is an 87-year-old gentleman who lives in a residential care setting. He has lived in the home for seven years and is receiving end of life care, as his health has been deteriorating. When Shamus dies, the senior staff at the home make a decision not to tell the other service users.

Explain the possible consequences of these actions.

If a person dies in a group setting, for example, a care home, careful thought and consideration must be given to how other people in the organisation will be supported. In addition to supporting the relatives and friends of the deceased, there will be times when other service users will need to be supported to come to terms with the death. Table 6.3 gives some suggestions for supporting individuals within a group care setting.

Table 6.3 Supporting individuals within a group care setting

When supporting individuals within a group care setting:	
Try not to overprotect other service users for fear of upsetting them	There may be times when service users have formed close friendships within the care setting. These people have a moral right to know if a person is critically ill or has died. Care staff often feel the need to protect other service users, for fear of upsetting them. Service users should be given the opportunity to express how they feel.
It is important that people do not find out the news by accident	Service users should never discover a person has died by accident, for example, by finding an empty seat where the person once sat. This may create feelings of mistrust and leave service users wondering what might happen when they die. Service users should be informed on an individual basis and in a sensitive manner.
Mark the person's life and death in some way	Some care settings will try to protect service users by carrying on as though nothing has happened. This can only serve to make service users wonder what will happen to them when they die. Will they be quickly forgotten? These service users will notice the person is no longer there and the fact that no one has acknowledged the death may lead to further upset. Careful thought and consideration must be given to the needs and feelings of the people within the group care setting. How would they wish to mark the deceased person's life? There are a number of ways in which care organisations can mark the life and death of an individual; for example, the organisation could write a tribute to the person, or observe a custom such as lighting a candle, saying a prayer or respecting a minute's silence, while some organisations may wish to open a book of remembrance. As well as indicating to service users that they too will be valued following death, these practices may also provide a great deal of comfort for the family of the deceased.
Find opportunities to talk privately with each person	Key workers should find opportunities to speak with each person in private. Service users must be given the opportunity to talk about their feelings and their relationship with the deceased person.
Encourage group discussion	If people wish to talk openly about the person's death, or death in general, this should be encouraged. It is often tempting to change the subject or suggest that people be 'more positive' about things. However, it may be important to them to be able to openly discuss and share their memories.

Evidence activity

 5.5 Describe ways to support others immediately following the death of the individual

You are caring for a service user who has died suddenly but peacefully during the night. Because the service user died suddenly, the relatives were not present at the time of death. The relatives had stated their wish to be contacted regardless of the time of day. How could you support the relatives at this time?

LO6 Be able to manage own feelings in relation to an individual's death

 Identify ways to manage own feelings in relation to an individual's dying or death

Healthcare staff tend to build relationships with those for whom they care. When an individual they care for dies, it is only natural that they will experience feelings of loss and grief. It is important for healthcare staff to acknowledge these feelings and not ignore them; otherwise they are in danger of becoming 'burnt out' and will therefore be unable to support others who are grieving.

Many organisations will have support systems in place for staff to express their feelings and work through their grief. Formal support systems include staff support groups, or one-to-one supervision with a senior member of staff. Counselling services should also be available for staff, if required. Support may also come informally from colleagues during a chat over coffee. It is important for any healthcare staff that talk about their feelings with family and friends to maintain confidentiality.

Some healthcare staff may prefer to express their feelings of grief by attending the funeral, or writing a letter of condolences to the family of the deceased.

■ Research and investigate

6.1 Find out how colleagues address their feelings following the death of a person they provide care for

Ask colleagues how they address their feelings following the death of a person they provide care for.

Evidence activity

6.1 Identify ways to manage your own feelings in relation to an individual's dying or death

Identify ways in which you manage your own feelings when caring for people who are nearing the end of their life.

6.2 **Utilise support systems to manage own feelings in relation to an individual's death**

It is essential that you recognise when you may need support. Observing and listening to the way that members of the care team support individuals may be of help to you.

Care staff should never be made to feel that they are being 'unprofessional' by showing signs of grief. If they hide their grief they are in danger of become 'burnt out', where the challenges of dealing with the demanding aspects of end of life care are unsupported, and the person suffers stress, anxiety and loss of motivation, which affects their personal and professional life.

There should be provision within your care organisation for staff to discuss and work through their grief. Referral to professional agencies should be available if a staff member is giving cause for concern.

Grief is an emotional response to loss; grief is an intensely personal reaction, but common elements are experienced in varying degrees by all bereaved individuals and are all normal components of the grieving process.

The time scale of the grieving process varies considerably, and may be helped or hindered significantly by the amount of support available for the bereaved to help them to explore their loss and continue with their lives.

Unresolved grief

Although everyone grieves differently, there will be certain parts of the grieving process that need to be worked through so the person can reach resolution.

Some people may not have had the opportunity to grieve properly. This could be for a number of reasons. They may have busy lives and lots of responsibilities. Other members of the family may have become reliant on that person to support them in their grief. This may lead to the grief reaction occurring sometime after the death. This is not necessarily a bad thing, as it is a release for the person's feelings of grief and part of the healing process.

Sometimes people may start to grieve but become 'stuck' at some stage of the grieving process. This may be in the initial stage, where the person remains shocked and in denial, and the person may remain stuck in this stage for years.

Sometimes people may carry on with their life but be unable to think of very little else other than their dead loved one. They may focus entirely on the dead person – affecting relationships with others as they, for example, refuse to clear away the person's room, clothes or other possessions.

Unresolved grief can affect the person's life, relationships and mental health. Help can be given in the shape of voluntary groups or care professionals such as counsellors.

Your feelings may seem unimportant, as you support people who are dying and the bereaved on a daily basis. Acknowledging your own grief and stress may make you feel guilty, that it is not you who should feel this way. However, to avoid excess stress and burnout you must look after your own well-being:

- **Take time out** – discuss with your manager about having a designated quiet area where you and other staff can go for time to yourself. You need to be clear about when this is appropriate and the procedures for letting others know where you are and how long you will be gone for. Taking time out at home may be helpful too.

- **Discuss your feelings with others** – colleagues, friends, family (ensuring confidentiality). Your manager may be able to arrange a support group within your care setting. You should be aware of counselling services, help lines, groups, etc.

- **Grieve losses** – acknowledge grief: cry if you want to (not in front of family); talk over grief with colleagues; mark the person's life.

- **Try to find ways to relax while away from work** – this will help you to reduce your levels of stress.

- **Rewarding oneself** – give yourself little treats and do what you enjoy. Never feel guilty because those you care for are going through suffering and feel you shouldn't enjoy yourself. Improving everybody's quality of life is important and that includes you.

- **Be aware of your own limitations** – you are not expected to know everything and cope with every situation. Know your limits and ask for support.

Evidence activity

 Use support systems to manage your own feelings in relation to an individual's death

What support systems are available to help you deal with your own feelings in relation to an individual's death or dying and how can you access them within your workplace?

Assessment summary

Your reading of this chapter and completion of the activities will have prepared you to demonstrate your learning and understanding of supporting individuals in the last few days of life. To achieve this unit, your assessor will require you to:

Learning outcomes	Assessment criteria
Learning outcome 1: Understand the impact of the last days of life on the individual and others by:	**1.1** describing the possible psychological aspects of the dying phase for the individual and others See Evidence activity 1.1, p.121
	1.2 analysing the impact of the last days of life on the relationships between individuals and others See Evidence activity 1.2, p.121
Learning outcome 2: Understand how to respond to common symptoms in the last days of life by:	**2.1** describing the common signs of approaching death See Evidence activity 2.1, p.124
	2.2 explaining how to minimise the distress of symptoms related to the last days of life See Evidence activity 2.2, p.125
	2.3 describing appropriate comfort measures in the final hours of life See Evidence activity 2.3, p.127
	2.4 explaining the circumstances when life-prolonging treatment can be stopped or withheld See Evidence activity 2.4, p.128
	2.5 identifying the signs that death has occurred See Evidence activity 2.5, p.128
Learning outcome 3: Be able to support individuals and others during the last days of life by:	**3.1** demonstrating a range of ways to enhance an individual's well-being during the last days of life See Evidence activity 3.1, p.129
	3.2 working in partnership with others to support the individual's well-being See Evidence activity 3.2, p.130
	3.3 describing how to use a range of tools for end of life care according to agreed ways of working See Evidence activity 3.3, p.132
	3.4 supporting others to understand the process following death according to agreed ways of working See Evidence activity 3.4, p.133

Learning outcomes	Assessment criteria
Learning outcome **4**: Be able to respond to changing needs of an individual during the last days of life by:	**4.1** explaining the importance of following the individual's advance care plan in the last days of life See Evidence activity 4.1, p.134
	4.2 recording the changing needs of the individual during the last days of life according to agreed ways of working See Evidence activity 4.2, p.135
	4.3 supporting the individual when their condition changes according to agreed ways of working See Evidence activity 4.3, p.135
Learning outcome **5**: Be able to work according to national guidelines, local policies and procedures, taking into account preferences and wishes after the death of the individual by:	**5.1** implementing actions immediately after a death that respect the individual's wishes according to agreed ways of working See Evidence activity 5.1, p.136
	5.2 providing care for the individual after death according to national guidelines, local policies and procedures See Evidence activity 5.2, p.137
	5.3 explaining the importance of following the advance care plan to implement the individual's preferences and wishes for their after death care. See Evidence activity 5.3, p.137
	5.4 following any agreed ways of working relating to prevention and control of infection when caring for and transferring a deceased person See Evidence activity 5.4, p.139
	5.5 explaining ways to support others immediately following the death of the individual See Evidence activity 5.5, p.141
Learning outcome **6**: Be able to manage own feelings in relation to an individual's death by:	**6.1** identifying ways to manage own feelings in relation to an individual's death See Evidence activity 6.1, p.142
	6.2 using support systems to deal with own feelings in relation to an individual's death See Evidence activity 6.2, p.143

Good luck!

Web links

Guidance for staff responsible for after death care	www.endoflifecareforadults.nhs.uk/assets/downloads/Care_After_Death___guidance.pdf
Alzheimer's Society	www.alzheimers.org.uk
Care Quality Commission (CQC)	www.cqc.org.uk
Cruse Bereavement Care	www.crusebereavementcare.org.uk
Department of Health	www.dh.gov.uk
Macmillan Cancer Support	www.macmillan.org.uk
Marie Curie Cancer Care	www.mariecurie.org.uk
National Council for Palliative Care	www.ncpc.org.uk
National End of Life Care Programme	www.endoflifecareforadults.nhs.uk
Princess Royal Trust for Carers	www.carers.org
Dying Matters	www.dyingmatters.org

7

For Unit HSC 3029
Support individuals with specific communication needs

What are you finding out?

Of the various skills that are needed when working in end of life care, none are more important than the ability to communicate effectively. Effective communication skills are vital to providing a high standard of care for people approaching the end of their lives and in supporting those who are close to them. It is therefore essential that staff have a good understanding of the importance of effective communication when supporting individuals in end of life care.

This chapter provides the knowledge and skills that address personal interaction and the use of special methods and aids to promote communication.

The reading and activities in this chapter will help you to:

- Understand communication skills in the context of end of life care

- Describe how to overcome barriers to communication.

LO1 Understand specific communication needs and factors affecting them

 Explain the importance of meeting an individual's communication needs

Communication is a basic human need; we all communicate and perhaps because it comes so naturally to us in our everyday life, it is easy to lose sight of its importance. We often assume that our natural communication abilities are sufficient. In end of life care, however, this is often not the case.

Time to reflect

1.1 Consider how often you communicate during the day

Think about how many times you communicate during the day.

In order to effectively support communication, it is helpful to have some understanding of what is involved in the process of communication.

Effective communication is indeed a two-way process. It involves an exchange of thoughts, feelings, views and emotions through the process of observing, speaking and listening. At a basic level, it is about getting your message across and understanding what others have to say. As a worker, you can provide a range of information for individuals who use services to enable them to understand the support that is available to meet their needs. You could ask the individual for their opinions about the provision available and encourage them to make choices.

Exchanging information is important for the workers; it allows them to develop their understanding of the needs of the individual, in order to provide the support they require and improve the quality of service provision. If the information exchanged is not accurate mistakes could be made, for example, an individual could be prescribed the wrong medication if the GP did not know they were allergic to it. If information is not exchanged, individuals may not feel supported and the workers will not be able to carry out their job roles as effectively.

Evidence activity

1.1 Explain the importance of communication in your work setting

Explain why communication is important in your work setting.

1.2 Explain how own role and practice can impact on communication with an individual who has specific communication needs

Communication is the process of transferring information from one person to another, using a method in which the communicated information is understood by those involved. Communicating with people who have a life-limiting illness may be difficult, because it may remind us of our own mortality and we may also be frightened of saying the wrong thing.

It is important to remember that a principle of end of life care is that people have a right to information about their situation so they can exercise autonomy. The principle of autonomy allows the individual to decide how much information they receive, if any, regarding their situation.

For communication within end of life care to be supportive, you will need to ensure you are communicating with the individual when and where they want to communicate. You cannot force someone to talk about their illness when they do not want to. Equally, if you appear to be busy or short of time, the individual will be reluctant to participate in any meaningful communication.

When communicating with patients and relatives about incurable and life-threatening disease, health professionals should remember to give attention to the environment and the physical comfort of all concerned. Standing in a corridor or a waiting room is unsatisfactory for everyone. Taking a patient or relative to a 'quiet room' to discuss painful and difficult issues has the advantage of signalling the importance of the meeting and the fact that the news may be bad. Many patients, however, prefer to be in their own bed space, with the illusion of privacy given by drawn curtains. This is because the bed and surrounding space is the patient's territory, where they feel most in control.

You will also need to observe the other person's body language and non-verbal communication, as well as being aware of your own. If you appear distracted or bored the individual will be reluctant to talk to you, so take care to ensure you are actively listening to them.

Effective communication requires the right conversations by staff with the right skills, taking place at the right time. It is important that they recognise and respond to the signs that someone is approaching the end of life and help them to start planning their future care. Staff need to create early and repeated opportunities for people to talk about these issues. They should be guided by the person on timing, pace and content, and respect the wishes of those who do not wish to discuss such matters.

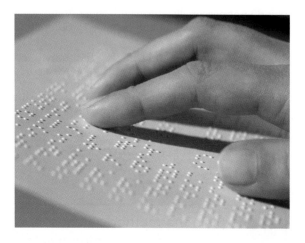

Figure 7.1 Braille

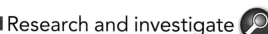

Research and investigate

1.2 Your view of your role in relation to communicating

How do you view your role in relation to communicating?

You must be sure that you give information in a way that can be understood by the individuals concerned. You must ensure that any specific communication needs are met. For example, people may require information in **Braille**, or to be communicated with by using signing. You will need to find out how to change the format of the information, or how to access it in a suitable format. Promoting choice and empowerment is about identifying the practical steps you can take in daily working activities to give individuals more choice and greater opportunities to make decisions about their own lives and the activities they wish to become involved in.

Key terms

Braille is a form of written language for the visually impaired, in which characters are represented by patterns of raised dots that are felt with the fingertips.

Make sure that the information is accessible by:

- presenting it in the most useful format
- making it available at the right time
- taking all the circumstances into account.

There are some aspects of empowerment and participation that are common to many settings and most individuals. If self-esteem is about how we value ourselves, then self-image is how we see ourselves and both are equally important. As part of empowering individuals, you need to consider how you can promote individuals' sense of their own identity. This involves making sure you recognise the values, beliefs, likes and preferences that individuals have and do not ignore or discount them because they may not fit in with the care system. A little thought and consideration can ensure that people feel they are valued and respected as individuals. For example, finding out how an individual likes to be addressed is important. Some older people, for example, like to be addressed as Mr or Mrs and using their title when speaking to them indicates respect.

When individuals want to make choices about their lives, you must ensure that you are doing your best to help them identify any barriers they may meet and help them to overcome them. When working with individuals in their own home, it is generally easier for them to make day-to-day choices for themselves.

Everyone is different. But we can tend to make sweeping generalisations that we think apply to everyone in a particular group. Therefore, in order to provide quality, empowering care, we must take the time to find out about personal beliefs and values and consider all aspects of individuals' lives. Although you may hold a different set of values or beliefs to the individual you provide care for, you must not impose your beliefs on them. You may need to act as an advocate for their beliefs, even if you do not personally agree with them. Value each person as an individual and be sure to be open to what others have to say.

The range of services and facilities that individuals may want to use is large and varied. Once people have the information on what is available, the next stage is to support them to make use of it. This may involve completing application forms or other paperwork, and you may need to support individuals to fill in any forms that are required to access their selected networks or services.

Evidence activity

1.2 Explain the methods a chosen individual uses to communicate

Choose one person – this can be someone you work with, a family member or a friend – and explain the methods they use to communicate. Are their methods effective, or is there something they could do to improve them? For example, if they have problems with their hearing, then a hearing aid may help.

 1.3 Analyse features of the environment that may help or hinder communication

The environment can be a barrier or a support to effective communication. It is important to learn how to improve and use your listening environment.

Awareness of personal space and positioning

Seating arrangements and the position of furniture should be considered carefully when communicating with others. Positioning chairs and other furniture between worker(s) and user(s) of services will depend upon the purpose of the intended communication. The height of chairs and tables can also influence communication.

For example, if the interaction is informal and between two people, sitting next to one another, with the worker mirroring the body language of the person could be most suitable.

If, however, the communication is to be of a more formal nature, then having a table at a higher level, with chairs placed near but on different sides of the table may be more appropriate.

Time to reflect

1.3 Consider what helps or hinders you in the environment in relation to communication

What helps or hinders you in the environment in relation to communication?

Comfortable, safe environment

A comfortable, safe environment may be created in the following way.

- Make sure that the environment is at the right temperature – not too hot and not too cold.
- Check the environment for any hazards and take precautions to reduce these risks before the communication takes place.
- Make sure the layout of the room is appropriate for the communication to take place.
- Make sure the environment has adequate ventilation – neither too draughty nor too stuffy.
- Check suitability of seating arrangements – some people prefer chairs with arms so that they can push up to get out of them; some may prefer softer seating, and others may prefer lower/higher chairs.

Respecting dignity and privacy

It is important to respect dignity and privacy. Make sure that you:

- Ask what name the individual prefers to be called by.
- Do not speak to the pusher of a wheelchair and by-pass the wheelchair user.
- Involve children in conversation – do not presume they do not understand the discussions.
- Offer choices wherever possible.
- Allow preferences to be expressed.
- Use a private room where appropriate.
- Do not discuss personal issues where others can overhear.
- Use passwords on the computer.
- Never disclose information over the telephone unless the identity of the caller can be established.

Evidence activity

1.3 Environmental aspects of work setting that contribute to or hinder effective communication

Take a look around your work setting. Which aspects of the environment contribute to effective communication and which aspects hinder it? Make suggestions for any improvements you identify.

1.4 Analyse reasons why an individual may use a form of communication that is not based on a formal language system

Non-verbal communication refers to the messages we send out to express ideas and opinions without talking. It has been said that as much as 80 per cent of our communication is expressed through non-verbal means. Non-verbal communication, otherwise known as body language, is a vital form of communication. When we interact with other people, we continuously give and receive wordless signals. All of our non-verbal behaviours, including the gestures we make, the way we sit, how close we stand, how much eye contact we make, send strong messages to the other person. For example, the way you listen, look, move, and react tell the other person whether or not you care and how well you're listening. The non-verbal signals you send may produce a sense of interest, trust, and desire for connection. On the other hand, they can generate disinterest, distrust, and confusion.

Non-verbal communication can be extremely important for individuals who are living with a life-limiting illness, especially if the ability to communicate verbally is limited. These people will rely on methods of non-verbal communication in order to make their needs and feelings known to other people.

We already know that communication is a two-way process. It is important that members of staff have a good knowledge of the power of non-verbal communication and use their observational skills, in order to interpret what the other person is trying to communicate through their body language.

The main elements of non-verbal communication are:

- tone of voice
- eye contact
- facial expressions
- touch
- gestures
- posture
- visual aids.

Tone of voice

The tone of your voice can say a lot more than the words you choose. Your tone of voice is capable of communicating many different things; for example, it may indicate that you are feeling upset, irritated, bored or angry. Care and attention must be taken when speaking to people, as they may become aware of your feelings through the tone of your voice.

There may be times, however, when you intend to communicate through the tone of your voice. For example, you may wish to let other members of the team know that you are annoyed about a certain situation, in order that an issue can be addressed.

Eye contact

Eye contact is an essential element of non-verbal communication. Eye contact can establish where your focus is. If an individual is talking to you and you are looking all round the room, it is very unlikely that you are giving the conversation 100 per cent of your attention. Equally, maintaining eye contact can convey interest and encourage the other person to become engaged in your conversation. It is, however, important to ensure eye contact remains natural. Blink naturally, as staring can be interpreted as being aggressive.

We can sometimes interpret thoughts and feelings through eye-to-eye contact. The eyes are particularly expressive in communicating joy, sadness, anger, fear or confusion. We can often tell what someone is feeling by looking at their eyes. Our eyes become wider when we are excited or happy.

It is important to keep your eyes at the same level as the other person's eyes, in order not to appear authoritative. This can be achieved by sitting down with the person.

Facial expressions

The human face is incredibly expressive. We are able to express countless emotions without saying a single word and, unlike some forms of non-verbal communication, facial expressions are universal. The facial expressions for happiness, sadness, anger, surprise, fear, and disgust are the same across differing cultures.

■ Research and investigate

(1.4) Facial expressions

In the space below draw expressions on the blank faces to show the following emotions: sad, happy, bored, aggressive, surprised, worried, pain, anxious.

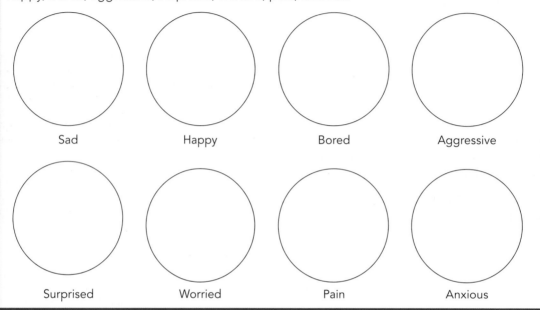

Facial expressions are often used to convey meaning when communicating. In fact, the face is perhaps the most important channel of emotional information. A face can light up with enthusiasm, energy, and approval, express confusion or boredom, and can also scowl with displeasure. A smile can show happiness and a frown can communicate annoyance.

Having the ability to read facial expressions is a very important tool when communicating with people who are nearing the end of their life. Very often it is easy to observe how a person is feeling through their facial expressions.

Touch

Touch is a very powerful means of non-verbal communication. We communicate a great deal through touch. Think about the messages given by the following: a firm handshake, a timid tap on the shoulder, a warm bear hug, a reassuring pat on the back, a patronising pat on the head, or a controlling grip on your arm.

Touch is an essential component of caring for individuals who are living with a life-limiting illness, and this can take the form of holding a hand, placing a hand on a shoulder or a hug. The use of touch can be reassuring and is a way of demonstrating that you care. Take care though, as not every person will respond in the same way to touch. If you do use touch, it is important to ensure that it is well received by the other person, as some people may feel uncomfortable being touched by others. It is also important to be aware of the importance of appropriate timing in relation to the use of touch. For example, if an individual is struggling with difficult decisions, the use of touch may cause the person to withdraw, rather than staying with the feeling they might be trying to express.

Gestures

Gestures refer to the hand and head movements or signals which many people use to emphasise what they are saying. Gestures may also help you to understand what a person is trying to communicate. There are certain common gestures that most people will automatically recognise. For example, a wave of the hand can signify hello or goodbye and thumbs up can mean all is well. Demonstrating an action may help people to understand when they find verbal communication difficult to follow. Equally, a gesture such as nodding your head can indicate to a person that you are listening. Although gestures can convey meaning, it is important to realise that the meaning of gestures can be very different across cultures and regions. It is therefore important to be careful to avoid misinterpretation.

Key terms

Gestures refer to the hand and head movements or signals which many people use to emphasise what they are saying.

Posture

Posture refers to the way in which you stand or sit. Your posture can indicate your confidence, openness and attitude. There are certain postures which can convey a negative attitude; for example, folded arms or crossed legs can send the message that you are being defensive, or are not interested in what is happening. A slouched posture may convey fatigue, poor health or low self-esteem. By contrast, a relaxed but straight posture is more likely to convey health, vitality and confidence.

Visual aids

Visual aids can be extremely useful when an individual finds verbal communication difficult. This could be because the person has little or no speech. Flash cards with pictures on them are an excellent example of a visual aid.

Research and investigate

1.4 Using visual aids

Which other visual aids have you used or heard of?

Listening

Developing effective listening skills is just as important as developing your speaking skills. Effective communication is a two-way process, and without effective listening skills, meaningful communication will be lessened.

Listening to people involves more than just hearing what they say. To listen well, you need to be able to hear the words being spoken, think about what the words mean, and then think about how you are going to respond to the person. You can also demonstrate that you are listening through your body language and facial expressions. For example, if you are yawning and looking round the room when a person is talking, you may give the impression that you are bored and uninterested. By shaking your head and frowning, you may give the impression that you disapprove of what is being said.

To be an effective communicator, you have to notice how other people respond to your communication. People react non-verbally both to the way that you are communicating with them and to the content of your communication. You can therefore obtain feedback through the person's body language. Indeed, this may be the only kind of response you receive from some people who are not confident enough, or who are too unwell to speak to you.

Communication difficulties can be very confusing and distressing for both the service user and for members of the care team, but there are many ways in which you can enhance communication through non-verbal means.

Evidence activity

1.4 Alternative approaches and methods of communication

Explain the alternative approaches and methods of communication a person may use and why.

1.5 Identify a range of communication methods and aids to support individuals to communicate

How body language and non-verbal communication aid understanding

We all need to communicate with other people. Communicating our needs, wishes and feelings is vital – not only to improve our quality of life, but also to preserve our sense of identity. We tend to think of communication as talking, but in fact it consists of much more than that. As much as 90 per cent of our communication takes place through non-verbal means.

Non-verbal communication is the way people:

- reinforce the spoken word
- replace the spoken word using their bodies to make visual signals, or their voices to make oral but non-verbal signals.

It is easy to take for granted – we are often not aware of our own non-verbal communication, but aware of that of other people.

Non-verbal communication functions to:

- convey our mood/state of mind
- convey interpersonal feelings
- support our verbal message if we are speaking
- provide feedback, assurance, etc. that we are listening.

Time to reflect

1.5 Observe and note a colleague's use of non-verbal methods of communication

Observe a colleague and make a note of the non-verbal methods of communication they use.

Body language is the non-verbal movement we make as a part of how we communicate, from waving hands to involuntary twitching of facial muscles. Facial expressions can indicate whether a person is feeling happy, sad, confused or if they are experiencing pain or discomfort.

Gestures can be very useful if an individual has difficulty communicating verbally. Thumbs up may indicate 'yes', 'good' or 'OK'. Thumbs down generally indicates 'no' or 'bad', while a hand being held up may indicate 'stop' or 'no'. It is important for healthcare workers to be aware of different cultures, as the meaning behind the gestures may vary; an everyday gesture used by one culture may be deemed rude and offensive to another.

Touch when used appropriately can be useful to convey sympathy and understanding or to let a blind person know you are there. It is important for healthcare staff to assess the individual's likes and preferences regarding touching. Touch is culturally determined! But each culture has a clear concept of what parts of the body one may not touch.

- Islamic and Hindu – typically don't touch with the left hand. To do so is a social insult. The left hand is used for toilet functions. It is mannerly in India to break your bread only with your right hand (sometimes difficult for non-Indians).
- Islamic cultures generally don't approve of any touching between genders (even hand shakes) but consider such touching (including hand holding, hugs) between same-sex to be appropriate.
- Many Asians don't touch the head (the head houses the soul and a touch puts it in jeopardy).
- Eye contact indicates a degree of attention or interest, influences attitude change or persuasion, regulates interaction, communicates emotion, defines power and status, and has a central role in managing impressions of others.
- Western cultures see direct eye-to-eye contact as positive.
- Arabic cultures make prolonged eye contact – they believe it shows interest and helps them to understand the truthfulness of the other person (a person who doesn't reciprocate is seen as untrustworthy).
- Japanese, African, Latin American and Caribbean cultures – avoid eye contact to show respect.

Proximity relates to space. We all have our own personal space that we do not wish others to invade. However, we let some people closer than others. It is important for healthcare staff to be aware of proximity and not to invade an individual's personal space, thus making them feel uncomfortable.

Research and investigate

1.5 Consider other aspects of space

What other aspects of space do we need to consider?

Posture: an open body that takes up a lot of space can indicate comfort and domination, while a closed-in body that makes itself small can signal inferiority. Copying the other person's body posture shows agreement, trust and liking.

Position: when positioning yourself it is important to ensure that you do not stand or sit at a higher level than the individual so that you are looking down on them, as this will put you in a position of authority and may make the individual feel inferior. Always lower yourself to the individual's level by crouching down or sitting. When positioning chairs for communication, try to ensure that they are facing each other or are at a slight angle. Try not to have tables or anything between you and the individual that can act as a barrier.

Paralanguage: is the content of your message contradicted by the attitude with which you are communicating it? Researchers have found that the tone, pitch, quality of voice, and rate of speaking convey emotions that can be accurately judged regardless of the content of the message.

Negative body language can make you appear defensive or disinterested. Try to avoid using negative types of body language such as:

- eye contact – depending on culture
- slouched position
- head down
- crossed arms
- sullen expression
- body turned away
- hand covering the mouth/face.

It is important for healthcare staff to be aware of all aspects of verbal and non-verbal communication when communicating with individuals. An individual who is in pain may deny this verbally. However, their non-verbal communication may indicate otherwise; for example, they may grimace and flinch away from touch; also the tone of their voice may sound flat. For someone who cannot communicate verbally, non-verbal signs may be the only indication that a person is experiencing pain or discomfort.

Evidence activity

Explain how you ensure that communication is accurate

Explain how you ensure that communication is accurate, whatever approach is being used.

1.6 Describe the potential effects on an individual of having unmet communication needs

As people approach the end of their lives, they and their families commonly face tasks and decisions that include a broad array of choices, ranging from simple to extremely complex. They may be practical, spiritual, legal or medical in nature. For example, dying persons and their families are faced with choices about what kind of caregiver help they want, or need, and whether to receive care at home or in an institutional treatment setting. Dying persons may have to make choices about the desired degree of family involvement in caregiving and decision making. They frequently make legal decisions about wills, advance directives, and Durable Powers of Attorney. They may make choices about how to expend their limited time and energy. Some may want to reflect on the meaning of life, and some may decide to do a final life review or to deal with psychologically unfinished business. Some may want to participate in planning rituals before or after death. In some religious traditions, confession of sins, preparation to 'meet one's maker', or asking forgiveness from those who may have been wronged can be part of end of life concerns. In other cultural traditions, planning or even discussing death is considered inappropriate, uncaring, and even dangerous, as it is viewed as inviting death.

The most obvious reason why end of life care is needed is to meet the needs of individuals diagnosed with a life-limiting illness. Everyone is entitled to good, high-quality end of life care. Unfortunately, too many people do not receive good palliative care and are left with unmet needs.

Unmet needs include:

- lack of, or little support for, family or carers
- lack of knowledge and information regarding diagnosis, prognosis and treatment available
- not being given adequate pain relief
- symptoms such as nausea, or side-effects from medication not being controlled
- emotional, psychological and spiritual needs neither acknowledged nor supported.

(1.6) Being listened to and understood

How would you feel if no one took the time to listen to you or to understand what you were saying?

Evidence activity

(1.6) Elise

Elise has a sensory impairment so it is very difficult to communicate with her. What problems, issues or anxieties might Elise have as a result of this?

LO2 Be able to contribute to establishing the nature of specific communication needs of individuals and ways to address them

(2.1) Work in partnership with the individual and others to identify the individual's specific communication needs

(2.2) Contribute to identifying the communication methods or aids that will best suit the individual

Traditionally, care was planned and delivered based on the medical condition and resulting physical needs of the individual. Each medical problem tended to have a generic care plan, as care plans were not tailored to meet the person's unique individual needs. Within the whole-person, or holistic, approach to care, the care plan looks beyond the physical need and will take into consideration the individual's:

- psychological or emotional needs
- cultural needs/beliefs and practices
- spiritual needs/beliefs and practices
- social needs.

A human's needs cannot be compartmentalised, as they are integrated and overlap. Being diagnosed with a life-limiting illness will probably have an adverse effect on all aspects of a person's life. Therefore, as a carer you will need to look at the individual as a whole and not just their medical condition. It is important to remember this throughout the individual's illness; even in the last few hours of life they will have more than just physical needs.

Research and investigate

(2.1) (2.2) Find out who is responsible for identifying a person's communication needs

Who else could or should be involved in identifying a person's communication needs?

Person-centred care is about providing care and support that is centred or focused on the individual and their needs. We are all individual and just because two people might have the same medical condition, for example, dementia, it doesn't mean that they require the same care and support. You will need to develop a clear understanding about the individuals you are working with. This includes their needs, their culture, their means of communication, their likes and dislikes, their family and other professionals.

Working in partnership with other professionals, colleagues, families and carers is an essential part of providing care and support. Person-centred care and support is about a whole range of people working together to improve the lives of individuals.

Partnership is all about the individual you are supporting and all of the partners involved will need good communication skills, sharing appropriate information and putting the individual's best interests at the centre of everything that everyone does.

Evidence activity

  Jeannie

You are working with Jeannie to assess her communication needs. How do you report on this and who needs to have access to the information?

Time to reflect

2.3 Information and support you consider would be useful in your job role

Write a list of the information and support you think would be useful in your job role.

2.3 Explain how and when to access information and support about identifying and addressing specific communication needs

If problems are identified with communication, there are a range of services which can be accessed. Never presume that you or anyone else can be heard, understood and responded to, without first thinking about the person involved. Check first to ensure you are supporting someone to communicate as effectively as they can, by working with them to overcome as many challenges and barriers as possible. It may be necessary to access additional support or services to help make communication better, or clearer. People may have problems in communicating with others due to:

- intellectual impairment, leading to problems comprehending and processing information
- sensory difficulties (hearing, vision)
- problems in understanding social interaction (e.g. autism)
- speech problems (e.g. articulation problems)
- others not listening and valuing what they are trying to communicate.

Many different professionals may be involved in supporting an individual with communication needs, but a person's motivation and efforts are equally important. Key experts likely to be encountered include speech and language therapists to help with communication problems, and advocates, interpreters and clinical psychologists to help with problems affecting mental processes and emotions.

Health professionals need to:

- take time and have patience
- value what is being communicated
- recognise non-verbal cues
- find out about the person's alternative communication strategies if verbal communication is difficult (e.g. their typical non-verbal cues, use of symbols, sign language)
- explain things clearly in an appropriate way (verbally and with pictures, etc.)
- be prepared to meet the person several times to build up rapport and trust
- use the knowledge and support of people's carers.

Evidence activity

2.3 Research and compare the key features of two different services

Thinking about the support and advice available, carry out research into two different services and compare their key features.

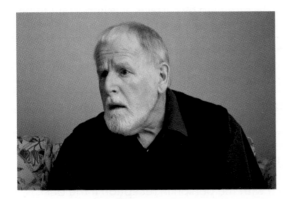

Figure 7.2 Poor communication may lead to confusion

LO3 Be able to interact with individuals using their preferred communication

3.1 Prepare the environment to facilitate communication

As well as your own actions and choice of words, careful consideration must be given to the environment in which the communication takes place. This does not just relate to the physical layout of the environment, but also other factors which can impact on communication; for example, lack of privacy and distractions from other people.

Environmental barriers could include those set out in Table 7.1

Careful consideration must be given to the environment, and how this can affect communication. This can be done in a number of ways. For example, you can:

- Ensure the layout of the room is appropriate for the communication to take place.
- Reduce background noise to a minimum – switch off the television or radio and move away from areas where other people are talking.

- Avoid interruptions – divert telephone calls and make sure other members of staff are aware that you should not be disturbed.
- Ensure confidentiality and privacy can be maintained at all times.

The environment must also be accessible for everyone. Healthcare environments can be adapted in ways that assist specific groups of people. For example, lifts can be installed that have sensors and a recorded voice to indicate when the doors are opening or closing, or indeed which floor the lift is on so that people who have a visual impairment can hear these messages. Ramps can be placed so that people who are in a wheelchair can access areas where steps are a problem. Reception desks can be lowered and signs placed in a position lower down on walls, so that people who are in a wheelchair can access the people and information they need.

Time to reflect

3.1 The effect of the environment on people when discussing confidential or sensitive information

Think of a time when you were discussing confidential or sensitive information. How did the environment make this more comfortable or more difficult?

Table 7.1 Environmental barriers to communication

Barrier	Consequences of barrier
Lack of privacy	Conversations should never be held where other people can hear them, as this is very disrespectful. Privacy is an essential component of confidentiality, and conversations that can be overheard may impact on the way in which the person communicates with you. In addition, interruptions from other people can make a person feel intimidated and unimportant. Lack of privacy, particularly, can be a problem within a hospital environment, especially when discussions take place at the bedside. Even when the area is screened by curtains, it is important to be aware that this does not make the area soundproof.
Poor lighting	A person who does not see very well may struggle to read written information in a dimly lit room. Equally, flickering lighting could distract a person, making communication difficult.
Distractions	These may include ringing telephones, televisions, other people talking, or even other members of staff seeking your attention.
Inappropriate fixtures and fittings	An uncomfortably furnished room which is poorly set out, for example, chairs too far apart or at differing heights, could make communication difficult. On the other hand, a person in a wheelchair may find it impossible to communicate with the person in reception if the desk is at such a height that the person in the wheelchair cannot see above it.

Evidence activity

3.1 Negative and positive environmental aspects of the area you work in

Draw up a plan of the area you work in, or socialise in, and identify positive and negative environmental aspects.

◼ Research and investigate

3.2 Using the wrong method or approach when communicating with a person and how you would correct this in future

Have you used the wrong method or approach when communicating with a person? How could you correct this in future?

3.2 Use agreed methods of communication to interact with the individual

The relationships between workers and service users, and also between colleagues, have a significant impact on the ability to provide effective care and support. Respect for each other can be developed through communication. Getting to know people by talking and listening to them will enable you to develop an understanding and awareness, which will lead to stronger relationships in the longer term.

Relationships are developed between workers and service users when they communicate effectively and appropriately, and trust is established. In order to maintain effective support and achieve success, each person involved in a relationship should know clearly what their responsibilities are and what the other person's expectations are. The targets for effective communication are to form a good working relationship or partnership where each contributor is valued. This involves:

- respecting individuals' rights
- maintaining confidentiality
- considering the person's beliefs and cultural views and opinions
- supporting individuals in expressing their views and opinions
- respecting diversity when individuals do not behave in the same way or have the same views as you.

Conversations are such common, everyday events that people often think they do not require any specific or specialist skills. Some interactions will be informal, such as speaking with friends or family members. Other conversations will be more formal; for example, having a conversation with a health specialist, colleague or employer.

Communication in work settings may be complex. This means that it may have several purposes. As a practitioner, you will need to be aware that each individual has their own way of interpreting what is said. Effective communication means more than just passing on information; it means involving or engaging the other person or people with whom you are interacting.

Communicating has to be a two-way process where each person is attempting to understand and interpret, or make sense of, what the other person is saying. Often it is easier to understand people who are similar to us; for example, a person who has the same accent as us, or is in a similar situation. The decoding equipment in our brain tunes in, breaks down the message, analyses the message, understands it and interprets its meaning, and then creates a response or answer. When a practitioner is speaking with an individual they are forming a mental picture of what they are being told.

Evidence activity

3.2 Explain how your setting ensures a person's preferred methods of communication are used at all times

How does you setting ensure a person's preferred methods of communication are used at all times?

3.3 Monitor the individual's responses during and after the interaction to check the effectiveness of communication

We have already established that some people avoid communicating with people who are nearing the end of their life for fear of not knowing what to say. There may indeed be times when there is no clear cut answer, but for the person who has asked the question, reassurance can be gained simply by knowing the question has been heard. It is therefore important that you:

- acknowledge you have heard the question
- demonstrate empathy and show the individual that what they have asked is important
- give the person your time and if you cannot answer the question, explain that you will ask a more senior member of staff.

When we find a subject difficult, uncomfortable or painful to deal with we use a technique that is referred to as 'blocking'. Examples of blocking when asked difficult questions include responses such as 'Don't let me hear you say that', or 'You have plenty of life in you yet'. These types of responses make light of the question and can deny the person the opportunity to express their feelings.

Time to reflect

3.3 Answering difficult questions

How would you answer the following questions? 'How long have I got before I die?', 'Has the cancer spread?' and 'Why am I not getting any better?'

A useful tip in answering a difficult question is to answer it with a question. By doing this, you are giving the individual time to think about what they have asked, and you can also give yourself a moment to think about your answer.

Evidence activity

3.3 Describe the action that your colleagues take while communicating to check that the information they give and receive is accurate and assess whether this is effective

Monitor colleagues while they are communicating. What action do they take to check the information given and received is accurate? Is this effective?

3.4 Adapt own practice to improve communication with the individual

Communication difficulties may isolate a person, making them feel cut off, so it is particularly important in a health or social care environment to overcome these difficulties.

The following adjustments can be made to help:

- self-awareness
- staff awareness and understanding of needs
- developing listening skills
- be aware of non-verbal communication, e.g. gesture, facial expression in self and others
- try to be aware of tone of voice
- be aware of personal space
- verbal, as well as written, instructions should be given
- if possible, give instructions one at a time
- good lighting is essential
- give positive encouragement
- be realistic in your expectations.

Communication issues might arise from a physical condition such as hearing difficulties or visual impairment, or as a result of a condition affecting the brain, such as Alzheimer's or a stroke. These communication problems may come on gradually, or could happen overnight, leaving you unprepared and unsure how best to communicate with the person.

You should also bear in mind that someone who has a physical or mental illness or disability may be affected by your own and other people's reactions to their condition. This could have an impact on their ability to communicate.

If a person's hearing or sight is impaired, body language and tone of voice will become more important. They may also need to learn new skills such as sign language or lip reading, in order to be able to communicate.

If a condition or impairment develops suddenly, you'll need to re-evaluate your methods of communication with that person. It might feel strange at first, but you might need to consider your tone of voice, how quickly you speak and how you use body language and gestures to emphasise what you are saying. It's a good idea to express this to the person you care for and find out what helps them, or makes your communication clearer.

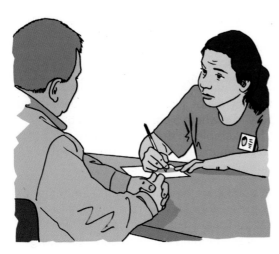

Figure 7.3 Listening

 Time to reflect

3.4 Your approach to communication and how you can improve it

Reflect on your own approach to communication. Is there anything you think you could do to improve it?

Adapting the environment can be done in a number of ways, such as improving lighting for those with sight impairments and reducing background noise for those with hearing impairments.

It is important to pick the right time to communicate important information to people. If, for example, a doctor has just told a patient that they have a life-threatening illness the patient needs time to take the information in. If the doctor tells them all about the treatment straight away, the chances are that the patient will not really hear much of what is said because they are in shock. It may be better to make another appointment for when the patient has processed the information and is receptive to hearing additional information.

Evidence activity

3.4 Following on from 'Time to reflect 3.4', ask a colleague or friend to review your approach to communication and compare their results with your own

Ask a colleague or friend to review your approach to communication. Did the results match your own? Are there areas for improvement?

LO4 Be able to promote communication between individuals and others

4.1 Support the individual to develop communication methods that will help them to understand others and be understood by them

Good communication, whether it is verbal, non-verbal or written must be at the heart of good practice when providing end of life care. Effective communication is essential for establishing effective and respectful relationships with individuals, their families and carers, and for assessments, decision making and joint working with colleagues and other professionals.

In order for communication to be **person cen-tred** and effective it must be based on principles which are **non-judgemental**, empathetic, **genu-ine**, **collaborative** and supportive. These principles are based on practices which involve active listening, reflection, respect, working in partnership, acceptance of other people's views and valuing the knowledge, experience and needs of others.

Key terms

Person centred: a person centred approach will place the person at the centre of all discussions and decisions.

Non-judgemental relates to an attitude which is open and not incorporating a judgement one way or the other.

Genuine: to be genuine indicates honesty, integrity and a commitment to be truthful.

Collaborative means to work together in a joined up way.

■ Research and investigate

4.1 Working with a person to enable them to develop their approach to communication

How can you work with a person to enable them to develop their approach to communication?

Ways in which principles can help to support communication are given in Table 7.2.

Table 7.2 **Ways in which principles can help to support communication**

Principle	How the principle can help to support communication
Non-judgemental	People may be concerned that they will be judged by others to be at fault for their illness. This is especially true where a condition could be perceived to be preventable, for example, in the development of alcoholic liver disease. A good communicator can help to relieve this tension by carefully avoiding judging the affected person.
Empathetic	Empathy is vitally important in good communication. Being empathetic when communicating involves the ability to understand another person's feelings and points so well that 'you could just about step into their shoes'. It involves hearing and understanding a person and expressing that you have understood.
Genuine	To be genuine indicates honesty, integrity and a commitment to be truthful. It also implies a capacity to communicate this truthfulness in ways that are thoughtful and sensitive to others' perceptions of events. This is about more than factual honesty or sincerity. It is also about earning trust under what can sometimes be very difficult conditions. This means saying what you mean and meaning what you say. Anything less could lead to a sense of betrayal.
Collaborative	Communication which is collaborative supports the notion that service users, their families and health and social care workers assume complementary roles and work cooperatively with other health and social care professionals. Together, these people share responsibility for planning and carrying out plans for the individual's care. Collaborative communication is about working in partnership with others; sharing values, agreeing goals and outcomes for the individuals they are supporting.

Principle	How the principle can help to support communication
Supportive	Supportive communication involves: • listening to what is being said rather than offering advice and guidance • communicating in a manner which is understandable to the recipient • showing that you are interested by ensuring good use of non-verbal communication • allowing the person time and space to talk • checking your understanding by summarising and feeding back, or asking for clarification or more information if needed • encouraging the person to speak freely, expressing their views and opinions • accepting that feelings may emerge unexpectedly and that it is OK for this to happen • enabling solutions to be raised and investigated • trying to identify the important aspects without being distracted by lots of little issues • facilitating the clarification of solutions and a timeframe for their implementation.

Evidence activity

4.1 Supporting communication

Explain how to support communication in ways that are non-judgemental, empathetic, genuine, collaborative and supportive. Explain how the actions you take ensure you communicate in ways that are non-judgemental, empathetic, genuine, collaborative and supportive when communicating with people who are nearing the end of their life.

 4.2 **Provide opportunities for the individual to communicate with others**

A person who is ill needs to talk, be listened to and be involved. All care workers should be trained to support and effectively communicate with the individual and their loved ones.

All communication should focus on the individual, their needs, preferences and method and style of communication. A full assessment of needs should be carried out and a care plan developed with the involvement of the individual.

All those involved in the care of the person should be fully aware of the contents of the plan of care and work together to promote effective communication.

When communicating with individuals it is important that you give them your full attention. This will ensure that you and they are able to communicate effectively, any barriers and difficulties are identified, and strategies are put in place to meet individuals' needs.

It is very important to interpret the needs of individuals and to motivate them to communicate. The way in which you approach individuals, and your willingness to help, will create an atmosphere in which they feel relaxed and able to communicate. Patience is essential, as people will feel uncomfortable if they are aware of being rushed, or feel that you are becoming impatient when they are trying to communicate. Provide them with alternative methods to assist communication, and seek the advice and support of key people within and outside your care organisation to provide extra support.

While encouraging people to communicate, you must remember that people should never be forced into communicating. They should be free to choose the use of gestures, symbols, drawing and the written word if they wish, providing this does not interfere with therapy or progress.

Some people may not wish to communicate at all. This may be due to a specific communication difficulty or a psychological or emotional reason. This should be reported so that the person can be referred for assessment by specialists.

Time to reflect

4.2 Consider the opportunities in your workplace for people to communicate with each other in a peaceful environment

What opportunities exist in your workplace for people to communicate with each other in a peaceful environment?

Evidence activity

4.2 Sienna

Sienna has been diagnosed with cancer but is very sociable. Her mother says that she should remain in her bed on the ward and not speak to others, as this will tire her. Do you agree? What action can you take?

In order to effectively communicate you must set the scene. This includes the following:

- Right place – ensure the person has a quiet place to talk with minimal risk of interruption. Ensure that the discussion takes place in private, where it cannot be overheard.
- Right time – wait until the person is ready and willing to talk. Asking them if they want to talk may be the encouragement they need. The dying person should always be allowed to decide what is appropriate.
- Observation – carefully observe the person's body language; their facial expressions, posture and gestures will give you clues about how the person is feeling and whether they are experiencing any type of pain or uncomfortable symptoms.

Always be mindful of your own non-verbal messages. If, for instance, you do not sit down, maintain eye contact and look interested in what the person is saying they will not be willing to communicate.

4.3 Support others to understand and interpret the individual's communication

We all need to communicate with other people. Communicating our needs, wishes and feelings is vital, not only to improve our quality of life, but also to preserve our sense of identity. If you need to communicate with someone, it's important to encourage the person to do so in whichever way works best for them.

We tend to think of communication as talking, but in fact it consists of much more than that. As much as 90 per cent of our communication takes place through non-verbal communication, such as gestures, facial expressions and touch.

Time to reflect

4.3 Consider the way in which you found out about a person's communication preferences when you started in your job role

When you started in your job role, how did you know a person's communication preferences? Who told you about them?

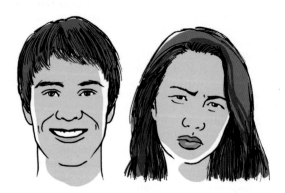

Figure 7.4 Facial expressions

Non-verbal communication is particularly important for a person who is perhaps losing their language skills. What is more, when a person behaves in ways that cause problems for those caring for them, it is important to realise that they may be trying to communicate something.

When communicating with others:

- Listen carefully to what the person has to say.
- Make sure you have their full attention before you speak.
- Pay attention to body language.
- Speak clearly.
- Think about how things appear in the reality of the person.
- Consider whether any other factors are affecting communication.
- Use physical contact to reassure the person.
- Show respect and patience: remember that it may take longer for the brain to process the information and respond.

Use your listening skills:

- Try to listen carefully to what the person is saying, and give them plenty of encouragement.
- If the person has difficulty finding the right word or finishing a sentence, ask them to explain in a different way. Listen out for clues.
- If you find their speech hard to understand, use what you know about the person to interpret what they might be trying to say. But always check back to see if you are right – it's infuriating to have your sentence finished incorrectly by someone else!
- If the person is feeling sad, let them express their feelings without trying to 'jolly them along'. Sometimes the best thing to do is to just listen, and show that you care.

Evidence activity

 Lizzie

Lizzie has just started working with you and needs to know the best way to communicate with each person. How can you help her to do this?

 Support others to be understood by the individual by use of agreed communication methods

Conversations are such common, everyday events that people often think that they do not require any specific or specialist skills. Some interactions will be informal, such as when speaking with friends or family members. Other conversations will be more formal; for example, having a conversation with a health specialist or colleague or employer.

Communication in settings may well be of a complex nature. This means that it may have several purposes. Practitioners will need to be aware that each individual will have their own way of interpreting what people say. Effective communication means more than just passing on information. It means involving or engaging the other person or people with whom the practitioner is interacting. The process of communicating involves various stages within a cycle.

Research and investigate

4.4 An interpreter

What is an interpreter?

Communication methods include:

- **Facial expressions** – a person's facial expressions can reveal a great deal about how they feel. They can indicate whether a person is happy or sad and also if they are experiencing pain or discomfort.
- **Gestures** – these are very important, especially if a person has difficulties with communication (e.g. waving a hand can attract attention) and restlessness can be a sign of pain, discomfort or worry.
- **Self-awareness** – it is extremely important that the care worker is aware of their own non-verbal message.

Evidence activity

 Explain what you understand by advocacy services and the benefits this approach may provide for people

Advocacy services have been accessed for several people you support. What is involved in this approach and what are the benefits for people?

LO5 Know how to support the use of communication technology and aids

 Identify specialist services relating to communication technology and aids

Using support services, specialist devices and alternative methods of communication

If you work in the health sector, you should understand the language needs and communication preferences of the people with whom you work. If an individual has difficulty communicating in English, or has sensory impairments or disabilities which affect their communication skills, specialist communication support may be needed. Learning a few words of another person's language, or developing some basic sign language skills, could help you to establish positive, supportive relationships with service users, their relatives or with colleagues.

A range of electronic devices exist to help people overcome communication difficulties. These include hearing aids, text phones, telephone amplifiers and hearing loops. Electronic devices can be used both to send and receive messages.

When interacting with people who have differing communication requirements, you will have to make use of skills to ensure you can communicate with the person. For example, if you are communicating with a person who has a hearing impairment, you should ensure you face the person as you speak. This will enable the person to see your facial expressions and read your lip movements. As you approach an individual who has a visual impairment, you should let the person know of your presence and whereabouts.

There are alternative ways in which some people may communicate within your organisation, and it is important that you have an understanding of these different forms of communication, in order that you can fully support service users.

Research and investigate

 Find out about the range of services that exist for people with sensory impairments

Visit the websites of Action on Hearing Loss (www.actiononhearingloss.org.uk) and the Royal National Institute for the Blind (www.RNIB.org.uk). Find out about the range of services that these groups provide for people who have sensory impairments. Produce a summary of the different forms of communication support that are available to people with visual or hearing impairments.

The following methods are commonly used to assist in communication with individuals.

Sign language is a visual means of communication, using gestures, facial expressions and body language. These signs are made up of the shapes, position and movement of the hands, arms or body and facial expressions to express a speaker's thoughts. Within Britain, the most common form of sign language is known as British Sign Language (BSL). BSL is a recognised method of communication for individuals who have a hearing impairment.

Lip reading is a technique used by some individuals who have a hearing impairment to interpret the movement of a person's lips, tongue and face. It is therefore essential when communicating with a person who has a hearing impairment that you look directly at the person who is lip reading and that you place yourself in a well-lit area when speaking.

Time to reflect

5.1

Have you used any of the approaches or methods discussed? Was it a positive interaction?

Makaton is a method of communication using signs and symbols and is often used as a communication process for those who have learning difficulties. Unlike BSL, Makaton uses speech as well as actions and symbols. It uses picture cards and ties in facial expressions with the wording, in order to make the word more easily recognised by those who have learning difficulties.

Braille was devised in the 1800s by a Frenchman called Louis Braille. Braille is used to communicate written information to people who have a visual impairment. Information leaflets and books can be produced in Braille. Each Braille character is based on six raised dots, arranged in two columns of three dots. There are variations of the six dots which represent all the letters of the alphabet, numbers, punctuation marks and commonly occurring groups of letters. Braille is simply designed to be read by fingers rather than eyes.

Remember, when communicating with someone who is visually impaired, it is important to emphasise your expression through your tone of voice and use of language rather than through gestures and facial expression, and that using touch to communicate certain emotions may be more appropriate.

Picture boards and symbols may prove to be useful when you are required to support an individual who may be unable to communicate verbally. There may be a number of reasons for this. For example, the individual may have had a tube inserted into the throat, or may have had an illness that has weakened the voice muscles. The individual may have suffered a stroke or other trauma and/or be living with one of a number of neurological diseases. These are all reasons that verbal communication skills may be limited. In such cases non-verbal communication replaces speaking, and communication boards are one common tool to help individuals to communicate non-verbally.

Assistive technology is used to support people with their daily living, including their communication needs. There is a range of equipment, including large keyboards and touch screens, which may spell or sound out words. Some people may use word or picture boards to support their speech. Others may use speech synthesisers, which replace speech either by producing a visual display of written text, or by producing synthesised speech which expresses the information verbally. Hearing aids, hearing loops, text phones, text messaging on a mobile phone and magnifiers are also examples of assistive technology.

Research and investigate

 5.1 Find out about other assistive technologies

What other assistive technologies are available?

Human aids are people who help in the process of communication. Examples include interpreters, translators and signers. Interpreters are people who communicate a conversation, whether it be spoken or signed, to someone in a language to enable understanding. There are many organisations that can provide interpreters for people who do not speak English, or for those who rely on sign language. These services may include social services, local communities, voluntary organisations and charities. When communicating through an interpreter it is important to ensure that you speak directly to the individual and not to the interpreter. Translators are people who change recorded information into another language. Signers are people who communicate using sign language.

Cultural differences can include social customs regarding dress, beliefs and values about family life, morals and religion. It is important to develop your knowledge and understanding of different cultures, to be respectful of differences and avoid projecting your own culture or background onto others.

Language differences can occur when the individual and members of staff do not speak the same language. Language may be misinterpreted or it may not be understood at all. You may need to engage the services of an interpreter or a translator. Written information should also be presented in a language which is understandable to the individual.

Assistive technology or adaptive technology (AT) is an umbrella term that includes assistive, adaptive, and rehabilitative devices for people with disabilities and also includes the process used in selecting, locating, and using them. AT promotes greater independence by enabling people to perform tasks that they were formerly unable to accomplish, or had great difficulty accomplishing, by providing enhancements to, or changed methods of, interacting with the technology needed to accomplish such tasks.

Providing support to meet the needs and preferences of individuals is a crucial aspect of your job role, which involves making sure that people are able to make choices and take control over as much of their lives as possible; this is also known as empowerment. It simply means doing everything you can to enable people to do this. Many people who receive care services are often not able to make choices about what happens in their lives. This might be due to many factors; for example, their physical ability, where they live, who provides care and the way services are provided.

Individuals who are unable to make choices and exercise control may also suffer from low self-esteem and lose confidence in their own abilities. There are other factors, which may impact on self-esteem and these include the degree of encouragement and praise we are given from important people in our lives, the amount of satisfaction we get from our jobs and whether we have positive and happy relationships with friends and family.

Self-esteem has a major effect on people's health and well-being. Individuals who have a positive and more confident outlook are far more likely to be interested and active in the world around them, than those lacking confidence and belief in their own abilities. Therefore, it is easy to see how this can affect an individual's quality of life and their overall health and well-being.

Providing an individual with information empowers them when they may otherwise have no control or power. Many people you work with may not have the information they need because they may not know the information exists, they may not know how to find it, or there may be physical or emotional barriers to gaining information.

When enabling individuals to access information about assistive technology it is important to consider the following:

* Make sure that the information is current.
* Go to the most direct source whenever possible.
* The information must be in a format that is understood by the individual for whom it is intended.
* Provide information at the most appropriate time for the individual, and as they need it.
* The information must be relevant and useful.

Evidence activity

5.1 Gina

Gina, who is visually impaired, needs support with her speech. What aids or adaptations will help Gina?

5.2 Describe types of support that an individual may need in order to use communication technology and aids

The term 'assistive technology' refers to 'any device or system that allows an individual to perform a task that they would otherwise be unable to do, or increases the ease and safety with which the task can be performed' (Royal Commission on Long Term Care 1999). This includes equipment and devices to help people who have problems with:

* speaking
* hearing
* eyesight
* moving about
* memory
* cognition (thought processes and understanding).

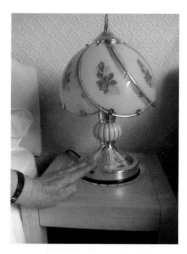

Figure 7.5 Touch lamp

Assistive technology ranges from very simple tools, such as calendar clocks and touch-lamps, to high-tech solutions such as satellite navigation systems to help find someone who has got lost.

Assistive technology can help by:

* increasing independence and choice, both for the person and those around them
* reducing the risk of accidents in and around the home
* reducing the stress on carers, improving their quality of life, and that of the person.

Selecting the right device is not always easy. Sometimes it may be that a non-technological solution is more appropriate. People react differently to various products. One person might find a simple recorded message that plays when they open the front door reminding them to take their keys helpful, while another person might find this confusing. Before you make a decision, seek as much advice as possible. Whenever you can, involve social services and the person's occupational therapist or GP in your decision, to ensure a tailored solution. If the assistive technology does not meet the individual needs and preferences of the person, it may be ineffective or even cause distress.

Research and investigate

(5.2) Determining the right technology or aids for a person

How can you determine the right technology or aids for a person?

Disabilities can sometimes make people wary of trying new things, adapting to changing situations or learning new skills, so it's important to find a product that really suits their situation, and their likes and dislikes. To overcome this difficulty, you may find it helpful to do the following:

- Aim to find solutions that can be integrated into the person's normal routine without being noticed, or with the minimum disruption.
- Involve the person in decisions about which product or solution to use, and take their opinions on board.

The level of support you may need to provide for an individual will vary depending on the circumstances. Your support can range from providing information to making all the arrangements to use the facility.

It is important that you encourage individuals to dispense with your support as soon as they feel able to manage independently. You should do this when you notice they are becoming more confident in their use of the technology. Gradually and appropriately reduce the level of support you give as they become more familiar with using the resource. It may take people a while to adjust to their new situation and they may need to make a few attempts before they feel confident to be left on their own.

Evidence activity

(5.2) Adreena

Adreena has been provided with several aids and adaptations but is not sure how to use any of them. How can you help Adreena?

(5.3) Explain the importance of ensuring that communication equipment is correctly set up and working properly

Technological aids and equipment can be used to enhance communication with people who may otherwise have difficulties. Some people may use word or symbol boards to support their speech so that a picture enhances the listener's understanding of what has been said. Others may use speech synthesisers which replace speech either by producing a visual display of written text, or by producing synthesised speech which expresses the information verbally. Hearing aids, hearing loops, text phones, text messaging on a mobile phone and magnifiers are also forms of technological communication devices. Voice recognition software can be purchased for any computer which supports the communication of individuals who find writing difficult.

Time to reflect

(5.3) Your feelings when a piece of equipment did not work or was faulty

Think of a time when a piece of equipment did not work or was faulty. How did you feel about this and what did you do?

It is important to bear in mind that communication can be affected by other factors in addition to the person's well-being. For example:

- pain, discomfort, illness or the side-effects of medication – if you suspect this might be happening, talk to the person's GP at once

- problems with sight, hearing or ill-fitting dentures – make sure the person's glasses are the correct prescription, that their hearing aids are working properly, and that their dentures fit well and are comfortable.

All equipment must be checked prior to use and on a regular basis once in use. If communication equipment is faulty or broken important information about a person's needs and well-being could be missed, leading to further anxiety or frustration.

When it works well, communication helps to establish trusting relationships, ensures information is passed on and understood, and offers choice and dignity. But all too often good communication is hampered by barriers. This can lead to misunderstanding, resentment, frustration and demoralisation, not only for patients/clients, but also for healthcare staff.

Evidence activity

5.3 Adreena's aids and adaptations will still not work

Some of Adreena's aids and adaptations are not working. Who can you ask for support and guidance?

LO6 Be able to review an individual's communication needs and the support provided to address them

6.1 Collate information about an individual's communication and the support provided

Every practitioner will need to be able to carry out assessment to the required standard; this may be daunting for those who are less qualified, so a team approach is supportive to all and makes the most of everyone's skills. In settings where there is a wide range of training and qualification levels, this is a challenging task and it is important to find ways of developing staff skills that keep everyone on board.

Practitioners are involved with the people they observe. They share spaces with them on a daily

basis and in this sense they are 'participant observers', rather than objective bystanders, in that they bring knowledge of the person and knowledge of context to that observation. In observing a person, the practitioner's intent is to construct a shared understanding of the person and how they cope with the environment and respond to situations.

Practitioners also bring themselves to the analysis of that observation, so the reflective process is crucial in developing the practitioner's awareness of being non-judgemental.

Observations are used to inform the person's progress and to:

- judge whether the overall aim of the plan remains appropriate to the person's needs
- analyse and evidence the impact of actions and services recorded within the person's plan
- ascertain if there are areas of previously unidentified or unmet needs.

■ Research and investigate

6.1 Find out how your work setting gathers and collates information on communication needs

How does your work setting gather and collate information on communication needs?

Person-centred planning is a way of helping people to think about what they want now and in the future. It is about supporting people to plan their lives, work towards their goals and get the right support. It is a collection of tools and approaches based upon a set of shared values that can be used to plan *with* a person – not *for* them. Planning should build the person's circle of support and involve all the people who are important in that person's life.

Person-centred planning is built on the values of inclusion and looks at what support a person needs in order to be included and involved in their community. Person-centred approaches offer an alternative to traditional types of planning, which are based upon the medical model of disability and which are set up to assess need, allocate services and make decisions for people.

Active participation is a way of working that recognises an individual's right to participate in the activities and relationships of everyday life as independently as possible; the individual is regarded as an active partner in their own care or support, rather than a passive recipient.

Person-centred care is a way of providing care that is centred on the person, and not just their health or care needs. Person-centred values ensure a comprehensive understanding of individual needs and the development of appropriate individual care plans for all individuals.

Person-centred values cover the total care of the person. To begin with the person is the centre of the plan, that is, to be consulted and their views are always to come first. It should include all aspects of care, including social services, health, family and the voluntary sector.

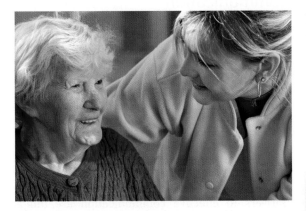

Figure 7.6 Positive support

Evidence activity

 Providing support to meet communication needs

Identify the communication needs of people you support and put together a short report on the needs you cater for. What support is provided to meet these needs?

6.2 Contribute to evaluating the effectiveness of agreed methods of communication and support provided

You will need to support individuals to review their progress and to identify the services and facilities which may need to be accessed to support them further. Identifying the options available to a particular individual and supporting them to assess the advantages and disadvantages of each will be an important part of your role.

You will also need to assess any risks involved with accessing any additional resources or services. For example, if an individual has to travel or is meeting with new people, there may be associated risks that will have to be assessed or managed.

Sometimes the options available may be disappointing for an individual. In such cases, it is good practice to prepare the ground in advance by encouraging the individual to consider all possibilities and to make contingency plans in case of disappointment. Be ready to suggest alternative approaches to problems, and new areas to explore.

If people are to make choices about their lives, they need information about the options available to them. There are many ways of making information accessible to people. These include not only the different ways of communicating mentioned above, but also ways of presenting information so that people can become more engaged in the planning process. At the moment there are many barriers which prevent the person at the centre of the planning process from being in control.

Research and investigate

 Find out about widely used methods of evaluating methods of communication

What methods of evaluating methods of communication are widely used?

Action for person-centred planning

For person-centred planning you need to consider the following:

- What method or combination of methods will be most useful to the person?
- How to give the person ownership and control over information about themselves.
- Allow enough time to produce information and resources.
- Link with other services to make sure that everyone is consistent in what they are doing.
- How to store and catalogue resources, so that they do not get mislaid.
- Your own training needs – do you need to go on a signing or ICT course?

There are lots of ways in which the physical space affects communication.

- Noise makes it hard to hear, and makes us tense and jumpy.
- Furniture arranged in a formal way, in lines or round a table, can make us feel inhibited.
- Big spaces make it hard to hear and see people.
- People entering and leaving a room make us feel our communication is not private.
- Uncomfortable chairs mean we don't feel at ease.
- Bare rooms mean there are fewer topics of conversation.
- Unpainted, dirty rooms make us feel devalued and worthless.

If we see things from the perspective of the person at the centre, it means we become aware of the importance of small changes. Choosing what to wear or where to sit, or what music to listen to may not seem very significant from our point of view – but these small changes can make someone feel effective and in control of a manageable part of their lives.

Evidence activity

6.2 Review the services provided for the communication needs of a person you are either supporting now, or have supported in the past

Identify a person you are either supporting now, or have supported in the past, and review the services provided for their communication needs. Are they sufficient? Are there any changes you could make?

6.3 Work with others to identify ways to support the continued development of communication

The purpose of communication is to get your message across to others clearly and unambiguously. Doing this involves effort from both the sender of the message and the receiver. And it's a process that can be fraught with error, with messages often misinterpreted by the recipient. When this isn't detected, it can cause tremendous confusion, wasted effort and missed opportunity.

In fact, communication is only successful when both the sender and the receiver understand the same information as a result of the communication. By successfully getting your message across, you convey your thoughts and ideas effectively. When unsuccessful, the thoughts and ideas that you convey do not necessarily reflect your actual thoughts and ideas, causing a communication breakdown and creating roadblocks that stand in the way of your goals – both personally and professionally. Reviewing the approaches used is critical to ensuring everyone is communicated with effectively.

Barriers to effective communication

Important and potentially difficult communications are frequently necessary with people who are receiving end of life care. This may include breaking bad news and treatment options, dealing with difficult questions and emotional reactions.

Despite your best efforts, you may sometimes find that you are unable to communicate effectively with another person in your work setting. There are a number of possible reasons why this might happen. Knowing about different barriers to effective communication will enable you to avoid potential difficulties and adapt your communication approach, where this is necessary.

Barriers to effective communication are things that interfere with a person's ability to send, receive or understand a message. Barriers include:

- tiredness or illness
- stage of end of life care
- language barriers
- cultural differences
- fear of dealing with strong emotions
- not knowing what to say
- environmental barriers.

Tiredness and illness

Fatigue, illness and stress can affect a person's ability to communicate. Many conditions can affect a person's ability to speak, understand and communicate, ranging from those which make speaking difficult to being completely unable to speak or understand speech. Conditions may include:

- **Stroke** – damage to the left side of the brain can lead to problems with speaking, understanding, reading and writing, described as aphasia or dysphasia. Damage to the right half of the brain can affect control of the muscles involved in forming speech, described as dysarthria. It can also affect memory and the organisation of language.

- **Alzheimer's disease** – people who are living with the symptoms associated with Alzheimer's disease, or indeed any form of dementia, will have problems with their short-term memory. These people may be unable to make sense of their environment and the people who surround them. They may forget recent events, and this will certainly impact on the way in which they communicate.

- **Motor neurone disease** – some people may develop weakness or wasting in the muscles of the face and throat, causing problems with speech and difficulty in chewing and swallowing.

- **Parkinson's disease** – Parkinson's disease affects the muscles of the face, neck and shoulders. Breath capacity is also reduced. Facial expression may be limited, giving the impression that the person has lost the ability to smile or frown. The voice is affected and can be weak. The muscles of speech are affected and speech may sound unclear or slurred.

- **Chest and lung conditions** – shortness of breath can affect a person's ability to speak in sentences.

- **Age-related decline** – age-related decline in physical abilities can make communication more challenging. A hearing loss makes it more difficult for the person to understand. Loss of vision will make it harder for the elderly person to recognise people. Some elderly people experience changes in speaking ability, and their voices become weaker, or harder to understand.

- **Depression** – may cause a person to become withdrawn.

- **Infection** – may lead to confusion.

- **Illness-related factors** – illness-related factors that might affect communication include pain, nausea, tiredness and lack of energy and loss of ability to focus and concentrate.

Time to reflect

6.3 Consider how to ensure that the support provided is consistent and continues to meet a person's needs

How can you ensure that the support provided is consistent and continues to meet a person's needs?

Stage of end of life care

Health and social care staff often find it difficult to initiate discussions with people about the fact that they are approaching the end of their life. Death may be seen as a failure by medical staff, who may not have received training in how to have such discussions.

A key challenge for all staff is knowing how and when to open up a discussion with individuals, their relatives and others involved within their care, about what they wish for as they near the end of their life.

Many people find it difficult to discuss death openly, let alone with a dying person. This is believed to be because people mistakenly believe that the dying person does not want to discuss the condition, or will be hurt by such a discussion. Good communication, however, is important at every stage of end of life care, yet barriers according to the stage of end of life care can present difficulties in communication.

Initially, barriers may be present due to the dying person believing their prognosis is better than that advised. The person may therefore feel the support of palliative care services is not required. Equally, the person may not want to be seen as a burden to others and may try to muddle through on their own.

The diagnosis of a terminal illness may be too painful or upsetting for the person, who may be unwilling or unable to discuss their needs or requirements for support. Equally, health beliefs and culture may prevent an individual from seeking the support of care services.

When an individual and their family are told of a life-limiting illness they may experience feelings of grief in relation to the anticipation of death. As a person experiences the emotions associated with grief, the individual's ability or want to communicate can affect the process of communication.

Towards the end of life, as the body's systems weaken, less oxygen is available to the muscles, the person becomes weaker, and more effort is needed to communicate. The person may become embarrassed, discouraged, depressed and irritable. Sometimes the person may sleep more, be difficult to arouse or become less communicative. This may be due to disease processes, medication, or the person's wish to withdraw from social contact.

The level of awareness and understanding can change frequently and unexpectedly, due to many causes; for example, the disease process, pain, lack of oxygen, tiredness and medication.

When a person becomes confused, this can be due to a decrease of oxygen to the brain and the person may not recognise familiar people, places, the time of day or year, etc., or they may hear voices or see visions, making communication very difficult.

Following the death of a person, relatives and friends will require varying levels of support. Providing quality care to people who are bereaved can be part of any professional's or volunteer's role and responsibilities. The period immediately following a person's death can be a very emotional time for everyone involved, including family, friends, staff and other service users. This is perfectly understandable and it is not unusual for staff to feel as though they don't know how to react or what to say. Under these circumstances staff may avoid engaging in communication, and this may lead to a situation where individuals are not adequately supported throughout their experience of bereavement.

Having professionals and volunteers that sensitively acknowledge death can be vital to people who are bereaved, as these people may have further questions they wish to ask about the causes and manner of the individual's death.

Language barriers

The United Kingdom is a multicultural country, with a mix of different ethnic groups and language communities. English may be a second or even third language for some people and may not be spoken or understood at all by others. Communication in written and spoken English may not be easy, or even possible, for people who do not understand the language. Similarly, people from different cultural groups may interpret non-verbal behaviour in different ways, thereby misunderstanding messages.

Even when speaking to people who speak English as their first language, careful thought and consideration must be given to ensure effective communication. Medical jargon and abbreviations only make sense to people with specialist knowledge. A person who doesn't have this specialist knowledge may not understand the message.

Sensory impairment is a term which is used when a person has a problem with their eyesight or hearing. People who have a hearing or visual impairment have different communication needs. A visual impairment may reduce a person's ability to see faces or read written signs and leaflets. A hearing impairment may affect a person's ability to hold a conversation because of the inability to hear.

Deafblindness is a visual and hearing impairment. These impairments can be of any type or degree and are sometimes called multi-sensory impairments (MSI). Some people who are deafblind may also have impaired speech.

Speech impairments, caused, for example, by an accident or a stroke, can impact on a person's ability to communicate. The individual may have very good understanding; however, they may have difficulty in making themselves understood.

Conditions such as cerebral palsy, cleft palate, Down's syndrome and autism can also affect a person's ability to communicate, both verbally and non-verbally; difficulties interpreting non-verbal communication may also affect communication if a person has autism.

A learning disability can affect or delay a person's intellectual development, including language and social skills. Many people with profound and multiple learning disabilities (PMLD) do not communicate using formal communication like speech, symbols or signs. But this does not mean that they can't communicate. If you work with a person who has a learning disability, you will need to be aware of their preferred way of communicating in order to fully support the person.

Some people have better communication skills and listening skills than others. We all process and interpret information differently, based on our own unique experiences. The level of trust between the individuals who are communicating can also influence the communication process. Communication is more likely to be distorted when people don't trust each other. Finally, stereotypes and prejudices can also impact on communication.

Cultural differences

These can influence communication. Culture is much more than the language spoken; it includes the way people live, think and how they relate to each other. Because different cultures have different communication 'rules', this can sometimes make effective communication difficult. For example, it is regarded as polite and respectful to make eye contact when speaking to someone in western culture; however, in some cultures this could be seen as rude and defiant. Within other cultures, children are not allowed to speak when certain adults are present, and within some cultures women are not allowed to speak to men they do not know.

Evidence activity

 6.3 Natalie

Natalie's care plan is being reviewed because her needs have changed. Who is involved in this review and what is their role?

Assessment summary

Your reading of this chapter and completion of the activities will have prepared you to demonstrate your learning and understanding of end of life care. To achieve this unit, your assessor will require you to:

Learning outcomes	Assessment criteria
Learning outcome **1**: Understand specific communication needs and factors affecting them by:	explaining the importance of meeting an individual's communication needs See Evidence activity 1.1, p.148
	explaining how own role and practice can impact on communication with a individual who has specific communication needs See Evidence activity 1.2, p.150
	analysing features of the environment that may help or hinder communication See Evidence activity 1.3, p.151
	analysing reasons why an individual may use a form of communication that is not based on a formal language system See Evidence activity 1.4, p.153
	identifying a range of communication methods and aids to support individuals to communicate See Evidence activity 1.5, p.155
	describing the potential effects on an individual of having unmet communication needs See Evidence activity 1.6, p.156
Learning outcome **2**: Be able to contribute to establishing the nature of specific communication needs of individuals and ways to address them by:	working in partnership with the individual and others to identify the individual's specific communication needs See Evidence activity 2.1, p.157
	contributing to identifying the communication methods or aids that will best suit the individual See Evidence activity 2.2, p.157
	explaining how and when to access information and support about identifying and addressing specific communication needs See Evidence activity 2.3, p.157

Learning outcomes	Assessment criteria
Learning outcome 3: Be able to interact with individuals using their preferred communication by:	**(3.1)** preparing the environment to facilitate communication See Evidence activity 3.1, p.159
	(3.2) using agreed methods of communication to interact with the individual See Evidence activity 3.2, p.159
	(3.3) monitoring the individual's responses during and after the interaction to check the effectiveness of communication See Evidence activity 3.3, p.160
	(3.4) adapting own practice to improve communication with the individual See Evidence activity 3.4, p.161
Learning outcome 4: Be able to promote communication between individuals and others by:	**(4.1)** supporting the individual to develop communication methods that will help them to understand others and be understood by them See Evidence activity 4.1, p.163
	(4.2) providing opportunities for the individual to communicate with others See Evidence activity 4.2, p.164
	(4.3) supporting others to understand and interpret the individual's communication See Evidence activity 4.3, p.165
	(4.4) supporting others to be understood by the individual by use of agreed communication methods See Evidence activity 4.4, p.165
Learning outcome 5: Know how to support the use of communication technology and aids by:	**(5.1)** identifying specialist services relating to communication technology and aids See Evidence activity 5.1, p.168
	(5.2) describing types of support that an individual may need in order to use communication technology and aids See Evidence activity 5.2, p.169
	(5.3) explaining the importance of ensuring that communication equipment is correctly set up and working properly See Evidence activity 5.3, p.170

Learning outcomes	Assessment criteria
Learning outcome **6**: Be able to review an individual's communication needs and the support provided to address them by:	**6.1** collating information about an individual's communication and the support provided See Evidence activity 6.1, p.171
	6.2 contributing to evaluating the effectiveness of agreed methods of communication and support provided See Evidence activity 6.2, p.172
	6.3 working with others to identify ways to support the continued development of communication See Evidence activity 6.3, p.174

Web links

Alzheimer's Society	**www.alzheimers.org.uk**
Care Quality Commission (CQC)	**www.cqc.org.uk**
Cruse Bereavement Care	**www.crusebereavementcare.org.uk**
Department of Health	**www.dh.gov.uk**
National Council for Palliative Care	**www.ncpc.org.uk**
National End of Life Care Programme	**www.endoflifecareforadults.nhs.uk**
E-Learning for Healthcare	**www.e-lfh.org.uk/projects/e-elca/index.html**
Action on Hearing Loss	**www.actiononhearingloss.org.uk**
Royal National Institute for the Blind	**www.RNIB.org.uk**

8

Care of a deceased person

What are you finding out?

None of us can fully understand the feelings of someone who is dying. Most people find it difficult to know how to support someone who is facing death. It may be helpful to try to think about how you would feel if you were in that position. It is important to realise that there are no right or wrong answers to this question and every person has different priorities. This is what makes the whole subject of supporting individuals through the process of dying extremely difficult. People are unique and so are their experiences.

Individuals may wish to have contact with, or be visited by, certain people during their final illness and may express a preference for who they would like to be present during their final hours, or who they wish to be informed of their death. These are obviously very sensitive subjects and should be handled with care. It is important that you fully understand your role, and appreciate that every person is an individual. It may be advisable for you to clarify your role and discuss these and other aspects with your manager, so that you feel better prepared to deal with these issues as they occur.

The reading and activities in this chapter will help you to:

- Understand how individuals wish to be cared for after death

- Identify the physical changes that take place after death and the effect these may have on laying out and moving individuals

- Understand your role in transferring the deceased individual in line with agreed ways of working and any wishes expressed by the individual.

LO1 Know the factors that affect how individuals are cared for after death

 Outline legal requirements and agreed ways of working that underpin the care of deceased individuals

It is important that care workers provide support for people in the final hours of their life. Every effort should be made to allow the person to express their needs and wishes and share their feelings and fears.

Many people will know that death is coming closer and will experience a range of emotions, including fear, and sadness. The way a person views death and what will happen afterwards will be influenced by many factors, including religious faith and their cultural beliefs, the experience of their illness and their personal circumstances. For instance, a very elderly widow, who is childless and has outlived most of her friends and family, may view death in a very different way to a young mother with school-age children. It may be far more difficult for the young mother to be at peace. However, do not assume that an elderly person is not frightened and has concerns they wish to discuss. Encourage the person to talk but do not push them. Be there to listen and provide comfort and pass on any wishes the person expresses.

A person may wish to talk to loved ones about the past they have shared, express their love and resolve any differences. People are different; while some may withdraw and not wish to talk about their impending death or any fears they have, others may wish to discuss their feelings in depth. However, it must be appreciated that families may have difficulty in discussing these issues and the person may need to talk to a health professional, minister of religion, solicitor or a counsellor.

All care must be carried out with the greatest sensitivity, preserving the person's privacy and dignity at all times. All requests for care must be responded to promptly and the person must never be made to feel they are a nuisance.

Time to reflect

 Being made to feel you are a nuisance

Have you ever been made to feel you are a nuisance? When did this happen and how did you respond?

For the person who is dying, there are many practical arrangements to be considered before death, such as making a will, and other financial, legal, and funeral arrangements. It is important that healthcare workers know where individuals can obtain information on such subjects. Individuals should be offered access to legal services, in order to sort out such things as property, finances and wills. It may be helpful to contact and arrange for a duty social worker to visit the individual so that legal matters can be dealt with. It can be a comfort for the person to know that their affairs are in order.

The person may wish to have a minister of religion or lay preacher to administer last rites. It is extremely important that any last wishes are carried out and that the individual feels reassured of this.

The signs of approaching death

As death approaches there are many physical changes that occur:

- decline in the senses – all five senses will begin to fail, although hearing may remain.
- changes in breathing – breathing may become noisy as secretions collect in the person's lungs and throat. This may be treated with medication. The breathing will slow and may become irregular with long pauses and deep gasps. This is referred to as Cheyne–Stokes Respiration, named after the doctors who first identified the condition.
- loss of appetite – as death approaches and the body begins to 'shut down', loss of appetite is very common. This should be accepted and the person should not be badgered into eating.
- decreased urine output – this is due to reduced fluid intake and organ failure.
- bowel and bladder weakness – this is caused by general frailty, increasing weakness and an altered level of consciousness, resulting in incontinence.

- declining levels of perception and lucidity – levels of consciousness and awareness will reduce and the dying person may misinterpret or lose touch with their surroundings, people or activities as they become disorientated to time, place and person.
- agitation – this should always be relieved and a peaceful and comforting environment created.
- profound weakness and increased sleep – extreme fatigue and low energy levels will cause a person to sleep for increasing periods of time.

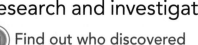

Research and investigate

1.1 Find out who discovered Cheyne–Stokes Respiration

Who discovered Cheyne–Stokes Respiration? Write a short paragraph about them.

Some people have very clear views about what treatment they would or would not like to receive in the final stages of an incurable illness. An individual who is fully aware and competent has the right to choose whether or not to continue with medical treatment, and no other adult has the right to make these decisions for the individual.

Within a document entitled 'Treatment and Care Towards the End of Life: Good Practice in Decision Making', the General Medical Council identified that some groups of people can experience inequalities in getting access to healthcare services and in the standard of care provided. It is in fact well known that some older people, those with disabilities and those from ethnic minority groups sometimes receive poor standards of care towards the end of their life. This may be because of:

- physical barriers
- communication barriers
- mistaken beliefs about what end of life care involves
- lack of knowledge among care providers, due to lack of training
- lack of knowledge about the service user's needs and interests.

The overall aim of equality, capacity and human rights law is to protect the rights of all individuals, not just those who access services. These laws also reinforce and emphasise the right that all service users have to be treated fairly.

The Mental Capacity Act 2005 is an important part of the existing legal framework, aimed at protecting the rights of individuals throughout end of life care. This piece of legislation came fully into force in October 2007 and applies throughout England and Wales. In Scotland adults are protected by the Adults with Incapacity (Scotland) Act 2000.

The primary purpose of the Mental Capacity Act is to promote and safeguard decision making within a legal framework. The Act does this in two ways:

1. By empowering people to make their own decisions, wherever possible, and by protecting people who are unable to make decisions by providing a framework that places them at the centre of the decision-making process
2. By allowing people to plan ahead for a time in the future when they may lack the capacity to make decisions for themselves.

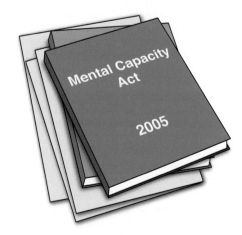

Figure 8.1 Legislation

The Mental Capacity Act has major implications for end of life care and advance care planning. It also addresses the rights of individuals to make advance refusals associated with care. This relates to the refusal of certain treatments, for example, a wish not to be resuscitated, or mechanically ventilated. This Act is aimed at protecting the rights of all vulnerable adults, and protects against healthcare professionals and others from making decisions for the person and overriding previously made choices. In addition, it takes into account the need for the person to be involved in decisions about their care, and is underpinned by five key principles. These are:

1. **A presumption of capacity** – every adult has the right to make their own decisions and must be assumed to have capacity to do

so unless it is proved otherwise. This means that you cannot assume that someone cannot make a decision for themselves just because they have a particular medical condition or disability.

2. **The right for individuals to be supported to make their own decisions** – people must be given all appropriate help before anyone concludes that they cannot make their own decisions. This means you should make every effort to encourage and support people to make the decision for themselves. If lack of capacity is established, it is still important that you involve the person as far as possible in making decisions.

3. **Unwise decisions** – individuals must retain the right to make what might be seen as unwise decisions. Everyone has their own values, beliefs and preferences, which may not be the same as those of other people. You cannot treat them as lacking capacity for that reason.

4. **Best interest** – anything done for, or on behalf of, people without capacity must be in their best interests.

5. **Least restrictive intervention** – anything done for, or on behalf of, people who lack capacity should be the least restrictive of their basic rights and freedoms.

The Mental Capacity Act 2005 is also backed up by a Code of Practice, which sets out best practice and covers an extensive range of guidance relating to specific scenarios.

There are also other pieces of legislation and guidelines that relate to people who may either lack capacity, or need to make decisions; and it is also important for health and social care workers to be aware of how these pieces of legislation may influence their practice when caring for people at the end of their life. Other legislation, codes and guidelines include, but are certainly not limited to:

- The Human Rights Act 1998
- The Data Protection Act 1998
- The Access to Health Records Act 1990
- The National End of Life Care Strategy
- The Nursing and Midwifery Council Standards of conduct, performance and ethics for nurses and midwives
- The General Social Care Council Codes of Practice (Note: The GSCC is to be abolished in 2012 and regulation of social workers will be carried out by the Health Professions Council, which regulates 15 professions including occupational therapists and psychologists. This is to be renamed the Health and Care Professions Council from 1 August 2012).

Human Rights Act 1998

The Human Rights Act requires public authorities to act compatibly with the rights set out in the European Convention of Human Rights. This Act came into effect in October 2000 and outlines 16 rights and freedoms that all individuals are entitled to. The Act makes it unlawful for any public body to act in a way that contravenes the rights and freedoms of people.

The Rights that have an impact on providing dignified care when supporting a person who is nearing the end of life include:

- **Article 8** – Right to respect for private and family life. This means that everyone is entitled to have their home and family life respected. Health and social care workers should always take steps to ensure the provision of care remains confidential and the person providing the care should have respect for the service user's right to privacy.

- **Article 9** – Freedom of thought, conscience and religion. This means that people have an entitlement to hold a belief or follow a religion and this shouldn't be restricted. This Article is relevant to social care because someone who belongs to a particular religion is entitled to have this respected. This may impact on the timeliness of care, including the times of visits, particularly during religious events and festivals. It will also impact on the purchase and provision of food, personal hygiene and care.

- **Article 10** – Freedom of expression. This means that a person is entitled to their own opinions, and should be able to express their opinions and ideas without interference. They are also entitled to receive accurate information. Within health and social care, this relates to the imparting of information. A person should receive adequate and accurate information, in order that they can make informed choices about their care and treatment. In addition, people should be listened to and their opinions acknowledged, accepted and acted on.

- **Article 14** – Prohibition of discrimination – This means that all people should be treated equally and without prejudice. Within health and social care, every person should receive the same level of care and should not be disadvantaged on the grounds of their gender, race, colour, language, religion, political opinion, origin, birth, sexual orientation, disability, marital status or age.

Data Protection Act 1998

The primary purpose of the Data Protection Act is to protect the individual's right to privacy when personal information is processed about them. This Act relates to the collection, use, storage, disclosure and destruction of personal information and applies to information that is held on computer, as well as written media, images and recordings. It is therefore essential that health and social care workers put measures in place to ensure the confidentiality and integrity of information held about service users. It is also essential that the information is only kept for as long as is necessary.

The Data Protection Act also gives people the right to access information that is held about them. For this reason, health and social care workers must ensure that written information is accurate, up to date, and free of jargon and abbreviations.

Access to Health Records Act 1990

Deceased people have the same rights to confidentiality as when they were alive. The Access to Health Records Act 1990, however, makes provision for someone who may be entitled to compensation to access records relating to the cause of death. This gives emphasis to the importance of robust and accurate documentation.

The national 'End of Life Care Strategy'

The national 'End of Life Care Strategy', published in 2008, is a comprehensive framework aimed at promoting a high standard of care for all adults approaching the end of their life; it identified a care pathway approach for the delivery of integrated care. The End of Life Care Pathway was developed to help those providing health and social care to people nearing the end of life. The Care Pathway identified in the strategy involves the following steps:

- discussions as the end of life approaches
- assessment and care planning
- coordination of care
- service delivery
- last days of life
- care after death.

The Care Pathway aims to ensure that high-quality, person-centred care is provided, which is well planned, coordinated and monitored while being responsive to the individual's needs and wishes. It is important that health and social care workers are aware of the strategy, in order that they can truly provide person-centred care which promotes dignity and choices for individuals who are nearing the end of their life.

The Nursing and Midwifery Council Standards of conduct, performance and ethics for nurses and midwives

The Nursing and Midwifery Council sets out the standards of conduct, performance and ethics that nurses and midwives must adhere to and apply within their work.

The General Social Care Council Codes of Practice

The General Social Care Council's codes of practice for social care workers set out the standards of practice that everyone who works in health and social care should meet.

Evidence activity

1.1 How an Act or Code of Practice impacts on your job role

Select an Act or Code of Practice and explain how it impacts on your job role.

 1.2 Describe how beliefs and religious and cultural factors affect how deceased individuals are cared for

Different ethnic/religious groups will have varying beliefs and practices. There may also be variations in the practices within the different groups. Healthcare staff may need to check with the individual or their relatives regarding practices; this should be done sensitively.

Buddhism

Buddhism is a tradition that focuses on personal spiritual development. Buddhists strive for a deep insight into the true nature of life and do not worship gods or deities. There are different schools of Buddhism and their practices will vary. However, one of the basic beliefs of Buddhism is reincarnation or rebirth. How a person is reincarnated depends partly on the frame of mind in which they die.

Most Buddhist patients will wish their condition and progress to be explained to them with openness and honesty, as this will enable them to make their own preparation for death. It is important that the individual or their relatives are able to contact a Buddhist monk (preferably of the same school) as death nears. Most Buddhists will know how to do this. They may give health-care staff a 'Who to contact' name. If the ministry of a Buddhist is not available, they may accept the presence of the Hospital Chaplain. If a Buddhist monk/minister is not present at death, they should be informed as soon as possible. Ideally, the body should not be moved before the arrival of the monk/minister, who will wish to say prayers with the deceased and this may take up to an hour.

Healthcare staff may perform last offices. It would be appreciated if the healthcare staff could speak to the deceased with respect and kindness, explaining what is being done for them. The body should be wrapped in a plain sheet.

Buddhists are usually cremated. There are no objections to post mortem or organ donation.

Christianity

Christians believe that there is only one God, whom they call Father as Jesus Christ taught them. Christians also believe in justification by faith – that through their belief in Jesus as the Son of God, and in his death and resurrection, they can have a right relationship with God, whose forgiveness was made once and for all through the death of Jesus Christ.

Christianity is diverse and encompasses:

- Baptist
- Catholic
- Church of England
- Church of Scotland
- Eastern Orthodox
- Exclusive Brethren
- Methodist
- Pentecostal
- Quaker
- Independent churches and missions
- Presbyterian
- Salvation Army
- United Reformed Church.

A dying Christian may wish to see a member of their clergy before they die to receive the sacrament of the sick. Healthcare staff may perform last offices. There are no objections to post mortem or organ donation.

Research and investigate

 Key points of a belief or religion

Select a belief or religion and identify the key points.

Hinduism

Hinduism is a diverse religion that was formed by the amalgamation of local faiths. The name Hindu was originally applied to people from India near to the River Indrus, on the borders with Tibet, Kashmir and Pakistan. This area is now considered to be where the original 'Hindus' came from.

Hindus recognise one God, Brahman, the eternal origin who is the cause and foundation of all existence. A Hindu's goal of life is to attain Nirvana, or oneness with God. Karma shapes one's current life and actions now affect this life and the next. Meditation rather than prayer is the preferred communication with God.

Many Hindus prefer to die at home. At death the soul may be reborn as another person, and one's Karma is carried forward. It is important for Karma to leave this life with as little negativity as possible to ensure a better life in the next birth. If the death occurs in hospital the individual's family may wish to call in a Hindu priest to read from the Hindu holy books and to perform holy rites.

Distress may be caused if the body is touched by non-Hindus. Therefore, close family members may wish to wash the body. Healthcare staff should respect the family's wishes. If healthcare staff perform last offices, the individual's hair/beard should not be trimmed. Cremation is preferred and usually takes place within 24 hours. Traditionally, the eldest son or other male relative prepares the body for cremation and makes the funeral arrangements. Post mortem is disliked.

Islam (Muslim)

Followers of Islam are called Muslims. Muslims believe in one God they call Allah. Islam is not just a religion; it is a way of life, as anyone who follows Islam accepts that their life will be spent in submission to the will of Allah, and obedience to the teachings of Muhammad, his prophet. Islam believes it is not enough to believe, faith must be put into action and practised, otherwise life is considered futile.

A dying Muslim may wish to sit or lay with their face towards Mecca. After death the body should not be touched by non-Muslims. Relatives or close family friends of the same sex as the individual will undertake the ritual washing.

Muslims are always buried with their heads turned towards Mecca. They are never cremated, as they believe in the resurrection of the body after death. Unless ordered by the Coroner, post mortems are forbidden.

Jehovah's Witnesses

Jehovah's Witnesses believe in one God (known as Jehovah), a spiritual being who created and controls everything. They believe that Jehovah created Christ, his human son, to redeem mankind from sin and death, and resurrected him to be our lord and saviour, but not as an equal to God. Beliefs are based on a literal translation of the Bible. All aspects of a Jehovah's Witnesses' life are guided by the Scriptures.

For Jehovah's Witnesses there are no particular rites and rituals associated with death and dying; a dying Witness patient may be grateful for a visit from one of the Elders of their faith. Healthcare staff may perform last offices. There is generally no objection to their doing so, as Jehovah Witnesses believe that when a person dies, their existence completely stops.

Judaism

Judaism is not only seen as a religion, but also a way of life. Jews believe God has chosen them and in return for his blessings they do their best to adhere to his laws. By adhering to God's laws and doing things in a way that pleases God, almost everything a Jewish person does becomes an act of worship.

Judaism can be divided into categories, which in turn may be subdivided:

- Orthodox Jews tend to be more traditional and observant of the religious laws.
- Non-Orthodox (includes Reform and Conservative) tend to make their religious observations fit into modern society.

A dying Jew may wish to hear or read psalms or prayers, in particular psalm 23. They may also like a Rabbi in attendance to help with their formal confession. Following death, it is preferred that the body be handled as little as possible by non-Jewish people, although non-Orthodox Jews will accept healthcare staff performing last offices if family members are not present. Unless legally required, post mortems are not permitted.

Rastafarianism

During the 1930s in the West Indies, descendants of a group of African slaves formed the Rastafarian movement. Despite regarding the Old and New Testament as scriptures, they do not class themselves as Christians. Rastafarianism is a personal religion placing emphasis on personal dignity and a profound love of God.

Rastafarians prefer alternative therapies such as acupuncture or herbalism. They are unwilling to receive treatment that may contaminate the body. However, those who visit doctors for advice are likely to accept conventional treatment. Visiting the sick is important among Rastafarians.

For the Rastafarian individual, there are no rights or rituals before or after death. Last offices are undertaken by healthcare staff. While burial is preferred, Rastafarians do not have a funeral ceremony; they believe reincarnation follows death and that life is eternal. A post mortem will only be permitted if the coroner orders it.

Sikhism

Sikhism is a way of life and in order to lead a good life, a person must do good deeds, live honestly and care for others, as well as meditating on God. Sikhs believe that human beings spend their time in a cycle of birth, life, and rebirth.

A Guru is a religious teacher in the Sikh faith. There were ten altogether, the last being Guru Gobind Singh, who started a new brotherhood of Sikhs known as the Khalsa or 'Pure Ones'. He instructed them to wear the Five Ks, which is a type of uniform that enables Sikhs to recognise each other as members of one community. The Five Ks are:

- Kesh – uncut hair, kept under a turban
- Kangha – small comb worn in the hair
- Kara – steel wrist band or bangle
- Kirpan – sword/dagger
- Kaccha – white shorts worn as an under garment.

A dying Sikh may receive comfort from reciting hymns from the Guru Granth Sahab. Usually Sikhs are happy for non-Sikhs to attend to the body, although many families may wish to wash and lay out the body themselves. If family members are not available, besides last offices, special consideration should be given to the 5Ks. They should be respected and left intact. If the family wish to view the body, staff should ask the mortician to ensure that the room is free of all religious 'symbols'. Sikhs are cremated and this should occur as soon as possible following death. There are no objections to post mortem.

Humanism, Agnosticism and Atheism

There are no special arrangements for Humanists, Agnostics and Atheists; after their death, health-care staff can undertake routine last offices.

Time to reflect

1.2 Specific needs you would like others to meet after your death

What specific needs do you have which you would like others to meet after your death?

Evidence activity

1.2 Lizzie

Lizzie is a Pagan. What beliefs and preferences might she have?

1.3 Identify the physical changes that take place after death and how this may affect laying out and moving individuals

It is important that you, as a care worker, are aware of the signs that somebody has died, as you may need to inform a senior person or a doctor. If you are in a more senior position, these signs will include:

- no response
- no pulse
- no breathing
- eyes fixed, jaw slack
- loss of control of bladder and bowels.

It is likely that during the period leading up to the final hours before death you will have got to know the dying person well and developed a relationship with them and their family. This can make watching the person in their final hours distressing. You, as a care worker, can do a lot to support and care for the dying person and their family. Creating a calm, peaceful and homely atmosphere

is essential. Critical observation during this period is a key task and a very important skill. This observation will help to determine how close the person is to death so that relatives can be properly supported and informed, and the person can receive appropriate care as changes are responded to quickly. In order to carry out critical observation effectively, the care worker needs to:

- be familiar with the person and their normal functioning
- observe for unusual signs and symptoms
- note changes in the senses
- report and record observations
- not hesitate to ask for support and guidance if they feel uncomfortable, unsure or fearful.

Research and investigate

1.3 Whom to ask for support and guidance

Whom can you ask for support and guidance?

Last offices

Last offices refers to the final care acts of washing the body after the individual's death and preparing it for removal. You should refer to your workplace policies and procedures regarding last offices, as procedures vary in different workplaces. However, when undertaking last offices healthcare staff should consider the following:

- **The dignity and privacy of the deceased** – speak to the deceased with respect; explain what you are going to do as if the individual was still alive. Do not talk over the individual discussing what you watched on TV the night before, etc. Privacy should be maintained at all times.
- **Respect for religious and cultural beliefs** – some cultures prefer family members or people of the same religious beliefs to carry out last offices.
- **Support for relatives and others involved with the care of the individual** – the support required will vary depending on people's needs.
- **Infection control** – wear Personal Protective Equipment (PPE) to reduce the risk of cross-infection.

- **Health and safety of others** – inform the mortuary staff if the individual has a pacemaker.
- **The safety of the individual's property** – follow policies and procedures to ensure the individual's property is stored safely. Check whether the individual has made any requests about jewellery, e.g. whether it is to be worn or given to relatives.
- **Workplace policies and procedures** – ensure you follow your workplace policies and procedures.

Last offices should not be undertaken until death has been confirmed and preferably be carried out within two hours of death being certified.

Last offices should be undertaken by two members of staff unless cultural and religious beliefs dictate otherwise. Wearing PPE the staff should:

- wash the individual
- comb and style hair
- clean under nails, trimming them if required
- ensure oral hygiene is completed and any dentures are replaced after cleaning
- check with senior staff before removing medical equipment; in some circumstances the equipment will need to remain in place
- dress any leaking wounds
- dress the individual in night attire, shroud or other clothes, as requested by relatives or the individual
- change the bedding, lay the individual on their back with head on one pillow, and cover individual with a clean sheet
- ensure mouth and eyes are closed
- place identification labels on the individual; check workplace policy regarding this.

Following the completion of last offices, health-care staff must ensure all relevant paperwork is completed clearly and accurately.

Relatives may wish to view their loved one following the completion of last offices and should be supported to do so.

Evidence activity

 Explain the key aspects of last offices and who carries this out

What are the key aspects of last offices and who carries this out?

1.4 **Identify diseases and conditions that necessitate specialist treatment or precautions when caring for and transferring deceased individuals**

All dead bodies are potentially infectious and standard precautions should be implemented for every case. Although most organisms in the dead body are unlikely to infect healthy persons, some infectious agents may be transmitted when workers are in close contact with blood, body fluids and tissues of the dead body of a person with infectious diseases. To minimise the risks of transmission of known and also unsuspected infectious diseases, dead bodies should be handled in such a way that workers' exposure to blood, body fluids and tissues is reduced. A rational approach should include staff training and education, a safe working environment, appropriate work practices, the use of recommended safety devices and vaccination against Hepatitis B. Examples of infection risks are given in Table 8.1.

Table 8.1 Examples of infection risks

Category of infection risk	Example of infection
Blood borne infection risk	Hepatitis B and C, HIV infection and AIDS
Intestinal infection risk	Dysentery, typhoid, paratyphoid. Profuse diarrhoea, food poisoning
Neurological infection risk	CJD, vCJD, TSE
Respiratory or airborne infection	Meningococcal meningitis, tuberculosis – open or closed (closed may become open during embalming or autopsy)
Contact	Invasive group A streptococcus. (Not MRSA unless invasive infection discussed with infection control)
Notifiable diseases	Salmonella, influenza, rabies, varicella zoster, measles
Viral haemorrhagic fevers and infections from travel abroad	Ebola, Marburg, Lassa, Crimean Congo haemorrhagic fever

There is a need to maintain the confidentiality of a patient's medical condition even after their death. At the same time, there is an obligation to inform personnel who may be at risk of infection through contact with dead bodies so that appropriate measures may be taken to guard against infection.

Personal Protective Equipment and personal hygiene

1. Persons who handle dead bodies must wear protective clothing consisting of gown/apron and gloves. Protective clothing or uniform must be kept separate from outdoor clothing.

2. When handling dead bodies, persons should not smoke, eat or drink and should avoid touching their own mouth, eyes or nose with their hands. Smoking, drinking and eating is forbidden in the autopsy room, body storage and viewing areas.

3. All cuts and abrasions should be covered with waterproof bandages or dressings.

4. Always observe strict personal hygiene, especially hand hygiene; this could be achieved by good hand washing or proper use of an alcohol-based hand rub.

5. Avoid direct contact with blood or body fluids from the dead body.

6. All efforts should be made to avoid sharps injury, both in the course of examination of the dead body and afterwards in dealing with waste disposal and decontamination.

7. Hand hygiene should be performed thoroughly after removing gloves and protective clothing.

Accidental exposure to blood or body fluids

1. In case of penetrating injury or mucocutaneous exposure to blood or body fluids of the dead body, the injured or exposed areas should be washed with a copious amount of running water. Minor penetrating injuries should be encouraged to bleed.

2. All incidents of exposure to blood or body fluids from the dead body, either parenteral or mucous membrane exposures, should be reported to a supervisor. The injured person should immediately seek medical advice for proper wound care and post-exposure management.

Evidence activity

1.4 Following standard precautions

What actions do you need to take when following standard precautions?

1.5 Describe the precautions needed when undertaking the care and transfer of deceased individuals with specific high-risk diseases and conditions

The care of patients presents a potential hazard of infection to healthcare workers with blood borne viruses through inoculation accidents with used 'sharps' and contamination of skin and mucous membranes with blood or other high-risk body fluids and tissues. Infections include Hepatitis B, C, etc., HIV and AIDS, Mycobacterium tuberculosis (TB) and some rare pathogenic Mycobacteria, Salmonella infections and Spongiform encephalopathy (Creutzfeldt-Jakob disease).

Since, without testing, there may be no way of telling who is infected with a blood borne virus, staff should practise universal precautions for all patients in their care.

- **Hand washing** – hands should be washed or decontaminated appropriately before and after each procedure. Cover cuts and abrasions with a waterproof dressing (no visible air-holes). If skin is contaminated with blood or blood-stained body fluids or other 'high risk' fluids, wash off immediately. Do not use an alcohol gel/rub, as this cannot penetrate organic matter.

- **Gloves and aprons** (non-sterile or sterile, as appropriate for the procedure) – gloves and a plastic apron should be worn for direct contact with any blood, blood-stained body fluids, high-risk fluids, or where it is likely that direct contact will occur; for example, in the course of performing procedures such as dealing with a blood spillage. Gloves must be discarded after contact with each patient and hands should then be washed.

- **Eye protection** – use mask/eye protection/full face visor, as appropriate to the procedure and where there is risk of facial splashing.

When removing contaminated linen use mask/eye protection/full face visor, gloves and apron as appropriate to the procedure and where there is risk of facial splashing. Procedures such as removing lines, for example, are associated with a high incidence of eye splash.

The routine use of waterproof cadaver bags is not required unless there is a specific infection risk, or there is leakage from the body which cannot be contained using absorbent pads, for example, from major trauma.

Transfer must take place to the undertaker or mortuary in a manner that prevents and controls the spread of infection. Where death has occurred due to a known, or suspected, infectious disease the body may remain infectious after death.

Research and investigate

(1.5) Find out about the correct procedure for the use, removal and disposal of PPE

What is the correct procedure for the use, removal and disposal of PPE?

It is possible for wounds, intravenous infusion sites, etc., to leak profusely after death; you should therefore ensure they are sealed with a firm dressing pad and waterproof tape.

Only wash those parts of the body which are grossly soiled. Attach identity bracelets to the wrist and ankle to ensure accurate identification of the body.

Viewing the body

Relatives and friends should be encouraged to view the body before removal from the care home. It is extremely difficult to arrange viewing once the infected body has been taken to the mortuary. It is inappropriate to discourage relatives from handling the deceased, especially if they have been caring for them while alive. It is best to advise against kissing or contact with any contaminated site.

Evidence activity

(1.5) Amira

Amira's relatives wish to view her body. What action do you need to take in relation to infection control?

LO2 Be able to contribute to supporting those who are close to deceased individuals

 (2.1) **Describe the likely immediate impact of an individual's death on others who are close to the deceased individual**

Although death is expected, many relatives may still be in a state of shock following the death and unsure of what to do or what happens next. They will need the support of healthcare staff at this time.

Loss, bereavement, grief and mourning

Definitions of 'loss', 'bereavement', 'grief' and 'mourning' are set out below

'Loss' is the disappearance of something cherished, such as a person, possession or property. The definition of loss also includes 'the act or instance of losing; the failure to keep or get something valued; the harm or suffering caused by losing or being lost; losses a.k.a. casualties occurring during wartime; destruction; and a measurable reduction in some substance or process' (http://dying.about.com/od/lossgrief/a/loss_define.htm).

The terms 'grief', 'bereavement' and 'mourning' are often used in place of each other, but they have different meanings. 'Grief' is the normal process of reacting to the loss. Grief reactions may be felt in response to physical losses (e.g. a death) or in response to symbolic or social losses (e.g. divorce, or loss of a job). Each type of loss means the person has had something taken away. As a family goes through a cancer illness, many losses are experienced, and each triggers its own grief reaction. Grief may be experienced as a mental, physical, social, or emotional reaction. Mental reactions can include anger, guilt, anxiety, sadness, and despair. Physical reactions can include sleeping problems, changes in appetite, physical problems, or illness. Social reactions can include feelings about taking care of others in the family, seeing family or friends, or returning to work. As with bereavement, grief processes depend on the relationship with the person who died, the situation surrounding the death, and the person's attachment to the person who died. Grief may be described as the presence of physical problems, constant thoughts of the person who died, guilt, hostility, and a change in the way one normally acts.

'Bereavement' is the period after a loss, during which grief is experienced and mourning occurs. The time spent in a period of bereavement depends on how attached the person was to the person who died, and how much time was spent anticipating the loss.

'Mourning' is the process by which people adapt to a loss. Mourning is also influenced by cultural customs, rituals, and society's rules for coping with loss (**http://www.cancer.gov/cancertopics/ pdq/supportivecare/bereavement/Patient/ page2**)

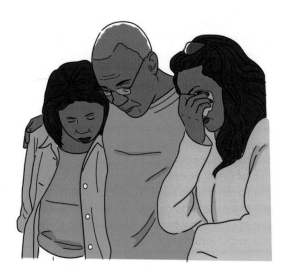

Figure 8.2 **Grief**

Factors that can affect the intensity and duration of a person's grief

People respond differently to grief. However, the following factors may influence how long and how deeply the grief is felt:

- how close the relationship was with the individual who has died
- previous experiences of loss
- the support networks available to the bereaved person
- religious or spiritual beliefs
- cultural beliefs
- age and gender of the grieving person
- the type of death: whether it was perceived to be 'good' or 'bad'
- whether the death was expected or not
- the condition of the body, whether the individual's body was disfigured as a result of disease or trauma
- the quality of the relationship just prior to death
- the need to hide feelings
- social support
- religious beliefs
- other life crises prior to death
- the person's perception of their loss
- the health of the bereaved person
- where the death took place: home/hospital/ care home/hospice
- anniversaries or other reminders.

No two people experience grief in exactly the same way, yet there are similarities in the feelings people experience when they are grieving. The feelings listed in Table 8.2 are not experienced in any particular order, except for the fact that shock is most often the first feeling experienced, and that people try to move through grief to arrive at acceptance at the end.

Table 8.2 Feelings people experience when they are grieving

Shock	Whether the death of a loved one is sudden or expected, people usually experience a period of shock when it occurs. When people are in shock, they feel neither happiness nor sadness. It may seem as if things aren't real. There may be a sense of disbelief. People have fragmented memories of things that happened when they were in shock. They may remember the faces of the people at the funeral, but nothing about what was said. There may be a sense of apathy, of not caring one way or the other about decisions that need to be made.
Anger	People who have lost loved ones will often feel intense anger. They may be angry at the person for deserting them. They may be angry at God for taking their loved one from them. They may be angry at the medical professionals for not being able to do more to keep their loved one from dying. This is a normal part of the grieving process.
Guilt	Feeling guilty is also a normal part of grieving. You may feel guilty for not doing more to encourage your loved one to seek medical attention earlier. You may have things you wish you had said before the person died. You may wish you had done more to help make them comfortable during the final days or hours of their life. Some people feel guilty because they have a sense of relief that the person is dead, and no longer suffering. Others feel guilty when they try to reinvent their lives; when they laugh or do something that they enjoy. They feel that somehow they are devaluing the memory of their loved one by starting a life of their own.
Sadness	This is the most common emotion associated with bereavement and can often be intense. Any little thing can trigger the tears, such as seeing something that reminds you of the person you lost, doing something alone that you used to do together, or having someone ask you about your loved one. People are uncomfortable with tears, yet tears are a natural part of grieving. It is OK to cry.
Hopelessness	When people are in the midst of grief, they often feel they will never get over it. They develop a sense of hopelessness, as though they are stuck in their grief. People do, however, get through the grieving process. Things will never be like they were before, but the intensity of the emotions will lessen with time. There is hope at the end of grief. People do reinvent their lives and find new activities and new people to do things with. Support groups have helped a lot of people to deal with their feelings of hopelessness. Grief is an almost universal experience. There are others who are dealing with these same emotions and can share their experiences with others.

As we grieve, our body experiences our loss as well and manifests itself not only emotionally, but also physically, cognitively, behaviourally and spiritually. However, grief can manifest itself differently in people, so not everyone will experience the same responses.

Physical sensations are often overlooked but play a significant role in the grieving process. Such sensations include:

- fatigue
- frequent headaches
- increased physical tension
- digestive problems
- loss of appetite
- flare-up of chronic or old medical problems
- crying
- tightness in chest
- tightness in throat
- 'heartache' (not to be confused with chest pain – always check it out)
- noise sensitivity
- breathlessness
- shaking
- palpitations
- feelings of emptiness in the stomach
- dryness of mouth
- shaking
- feeling weak.

Emotional response: following a significant loss, we are overcome with a number of feelings; in addition to those identified in Table 8.2, for example, we may experience:

- anxiety
- abandonment
- relief
- fear
- irritability
- loneliness
- confusion
- freedom
- depression
- feeling overwhelmed
- numbness
- feelings of powerlessness or helplessness
- yearning.

Cognitive changes: there are many different thought patterns that mark the experience of grief; they are all a part of normal grieving and may include:

- difficulty concentrating
- memory impairment

- decreased ability to problem solve, calculate or make decisions
- absent-mindedness
- increased daydreams and/or night dreams or nightmares
- being preoccupied with thoughts of the deceased
- hearing, seeing or sensing the presence of the deceased
- disbelief
- forgetfulness
- hallucinations: see, smell, or hear the person, particularly in familiar settings
- need to retell the details of the loss again and again.

Behavioural changes: a number of specific behaviours are frequently associated with normal grief reactions. The behaviours are commonly reported after a loss and usually correct themselves over time:

- withdrawal from family, friends, peers
- silence
- talkativeness
- lack of interest in anything that usually satisfies
- over-interest in things that distract
- never wanting to be alone
- carrying treasured objects of the deceased
- avoiding reminders of the deceased
- not talking about the death
- other changes in behaviour that you or others notice
- absent-minded behaviour
- searching or calling out for the deceased
- changes in sleep pattern, inability to sleep, early morning awakening
- changes in eating habits
- crying
- restlessness
- over-activity.

Spiritual re-evaluation: many people will start to re-evaluate their spiritual beliefs. They may:

- find comfort in spiritual and religious beliefs
- turn to religion
- question beliefs
- question values
- ask 'why' questions
- not find meaning in things at this time
- re-evaluate their life
- change their church habits

- change their relationships with family, friends, co-workers
- change their relationship to oneself.

Unresolved or complicated grief

Grief impacts each person differently and prolonged grieving is not unusual. For some, during the first few months it can seem as though the feelings of grief are overwhelming and will forever change all aspects of their life. While there is no set formula for how long it takes to move through the grieving process, it usually takes a year after the death of a loved one to move through a wide range of grief-associated emotions and begin to come to terms with the loss. Although there is no set time-frame some people may come to terms with their loss quicker than others.

Unfortunately, some individuals' response to significant loss remains stuck in an unresolved and long-lasting state. Sometimes this is referred to as complicated grief.

Time to reflect

2.1 Experience of personal grief, your feelings and the support you accessed

If you have experienced personal grief what feelings did you have? What support, if any, did you access?

Reasons people may experience unresolved grief include:

- Not having had the opportunity to grieve properly – this may be because they lead busy lives and have been too busy to grieve, or other family members are dependent on them for support with their own grief.
- Grief process is started but not completed – this may be because the person has become stuck in one stage or another.
- Carry on with life, but being unable to think of very little else but their dead loved one.
- Avoidance of grief – this may be because they are unable to cope with the pain of grief.

Enduring and hidden grief

Enduring grief is a type of grief that will never go away, but does not necessarily paralyse the person in the same way as someone 'stuck' in disbelief or denial. Some move on with their lives though their grief does not subside; instead it endures.

Hidden grief is a solitary grief that is not visible to others. Some people may hide their grief from others because of other people's responses to displays of grief. Some may feel it is unacceptable to display their grief due to the nature of their relationship with the deceased individual. Others hide their grief because they do not know how to express their grief. People who hide their grief for whatever reason will grieve alone and unsupported as others perceive they are coping.

The support healthcare staff can offer the bereaved

Healthcare staff providing end of life care to an individual with a life-threatening illness will also have been supporting the individual's relatives, as discussed previously. This support does not stop just because the individual has died. As healthcare staff you can offer the bereaved emotional, practical, informational or spiritual support.

This support can be achieved by:

- providing a quiet area where the bereaved can gather their thoughts or talk to you
- listening to the person, using active listening skills
- allowing the bereaved time to express their feelings without being rushed
- showing empathy, concern and compassion
- touching to comfort an individual; however, touch is not always appropriate and should be used with caution
- making refreshments
- greeting other relatives as they arrive
- contacting and informing other relatives
- arranging transport to take the bereaved home if death occurred in a care environment
- providing factual information in a manner the bereaved will understand; you may need to repeat the information or write it down
- respecting the beliefs of the bereaved
- contacting a religious leader appropriate to their religious beliefs
- treating the bereaved with respect and sensitivity
- validating the bereaved person's feelings
- informing the bereaved regarding collection of death certificate, viewing deceased, etc.
- providing information regarding bereavement support if required.

It is important that as a healthcare worker you recognise your own limitations and ability to support the bereaved. It may be that you feel unable to support the bereaved person to meet their needs. If this happens, seek advice and guidance from your manager.

There are times when the bereaved will require more support than you and your workplace are able to provide. Additional support may include:

- bereavement counselling
- social services
- charitable organisations.

You will be able to support the bereaved to access the additional support by referring them to the appropriate service, or providing them with relevant information regarding the services. Remember the support you as a healthcare worker can provide will not only depend on your qualifications, knowledge and experience, but also on the needs of the bereaved individual.

Grief work

The psychological process of coping with a significant loss is called 'grief work'. Just as the body heals if certain conditions are met, so will the mind. The goals of grief work involve working through the tasks and emotions of each stage of grief.

In his book, *Grief Counseling and Grief Therapy*, William Worden (1991) identified four stages of grief and the tasks of mourning an individual has to progress through so that they can complete the grieving process. Grief is deeply personal. Although four stages and tasks of grief have been identified, everyone will move through them differently. People may move through the phases quickly or slowly; some may move through them in a different order; others may skip a phase or task altogether. However, people should move through the grieving process in a way that will be the right way for them.

The stages of grief are shown in Table 8.3.

Table 8.3 Stages of grief

Stage	Feelings people experience
Stage 1: numbness	This is the phase immediately following a loss. The grieving person feels numb, which is a defence mechanism that allows them to survive emotionally.
Stage 2: pining and searching	The grieving person longing or pining for the deceased to return characterises this stage. The bereaved person will be preoccupied with thoughts of the person they have lost and may be desperate to see the person again. This may lead the grieving person to start searching for their loved one. The searching may involve searching for memories or reminders of the person they have lost. They may even search in crowds and imagine they see their loved one. Many emotions are expressed during this time and may include weeping, anger, anxiety, and confusion.
Stage 3: disorganisation and despair	The grieving person now desires to withdraw and disengage from others and activities they regularly enjoyed. Feelings of pining and yearning become less intense, while periods of apathy, meaning an absence of emotion, and despair increase.
Stage 4: reorganisation and recovery	In this final phase the grieving person begins to return to a new state of 'normal'. Weight loss experienced during intense grieving may be regained, energy levels increase, and an interest to return to activities of enjoyment returns. Grief never ends but thoughts of sadness and despair are diminished, while positive memories of the deceased take over.

There are specific tasks of mourning that need to be accomplished in order for mourning to be completed. The concept of tasks implies that effort on the part of the individual is required. These tasks are shown in Table 8.4.

Table 8.4 Specific tasks of mourning

Task	Effort required by the individual
Task 1: to accept the reality of the loss	Following a death, there is normally a sense that it has not happened even when the death is expected. The first task of mourning is to come to terms with the reality that the person is dead and will not return. Often the bereaved refuse to face the reality of the loss, and may go through a process of not believing, and pretending that the person is not really dead. A bereaved person will not be able to cope with the emotional impact of the loss until first coming to terms with the fact that the loss has happened.
Task 2: to work through the pain of grief	This includes the literal physical pain that many people experience, as well as the emotional and behavioural pain associated with the loss. The intensity of the pain varies from person to person and is not always felt in the same way; nevertheless, it is impossible to lose someone you love without suffering some degree of pain. If the pain is not worked through, it will manifest in some other symptom or behaviour. The bereaved may deny the pain or hinder the grieving process by avoiding painful thoughts, by idealising the dead or by moving to a new area where there are no painful memories of the deceased.
Task 3: to adjust to an environment in which the deceased is missing	Adjusting to the new environment means different things to different people, and greatly depends on the relationship with and the role of the deceased. The bereaved person often only becomes aware of the roles the deceased played some time after the loss has occurred. They are then faced with the need to develop new skills. Many resent having to develop new skills to cope with the changed situation. If attempts to fulfil the roles previously carried out by the deceased fail, a reduction in self-esteem can result. Not adjusting to the loss, not developing the new skills needed and remaining helpless, or by withdrawing from the environment and not facing up to what is required of them, is to avoid this task.
Task 4: to emotionally relocate the deceased and move on with life	The final task is to effect emotional withdrawal from the deceased, in order to make new relationships. The incompletion of this task would be in not loving – by holding on to the past attachment rather than going forward and forming new ones. For some, loss is so painful they vow never to love again.

How to support people during the various stages of their bereavement

The bereaved will require varying degrees of support while working through the stages of grief. The support you provide can be given at any stage and is not confined to any one particular stage.

Healthcare workers can support the bereaved through the stages of grief by:

- being there and listening to them in an accepting and non-judgemental way
- not offering solutions or colluding with them
- showing them you are listening and understand something of what they are going through
- allowing them to talk about the deceased as often as they want, mention the deceased by name, talk about the special, endearing qualities of what they have lost
- allowing silences during conversation; silences are useful thinking time
- being available to listen or help with whatever else seems needed at the time
- allowing them to express as much unhappiness as they are feeling at that moment and are willing to share
- letting your genuine concern and caring show
- being familiar with your own feelings about loss and grief: know your own fears and difficult feelings
- offering reassurance about the normality and duration of grief, and about the future
- accepting their anger as part of their grief; do not take it personally
- recognising that your feelings may reflect how they feel: feelings of helplessness, hopelessness, frustration or anger may be what the other person is feeling
- accepting that you cannot make them feel better: you are still doing something useful, even if it does not feel like it
- encouraging them to be patient with themselves, not expect too much of themselves
- reassuring them that they did everything that they could
- letting the bereaved progress through each stage at their own rate – do not rush them
- giving positive feedback if you feel they are making progress through a stage
- referring them to a support group or bereavement counsellor if additional support is required.

Evidence activity

 2.1 Summarise the key points of the stages of bereavement

Write a summary of the key points of the stages of bereavement.

2.2 **Support others immediately following the death of the individual in ways that:**
- **reduce their distress**
- **respect the deceased individual**

As a healthcare worker, following the death of an individual you can support the relatives in the following ways:

- Contact relatives and friends in accordance with previously ascertained wishes.
- Be prepared for different responses to death.
- Allow bereaved people to sit by the deceased person for as long as they wish.
- Offer refreshments and provide a quiet space.
- Ensure that a key member of staff is available.
- Ensure meetings are free from interruption.
- Provide practical information at an appropriate moment.
- Collect and present the person's possessions in a thoughtful manner.
- Ask a relative who is alone if there is anyone you can contact for them.

If a person dies overnight some relatives may choose to go home. Every single person has their own way of coping with the situation. Relatives may express a wish to be contacted at the time of death. It is therefore very important that an accurate record be kept in the individual's notes. This should include:

- next of kin details
- telephone number and address details of persons to be contacted.

It is vital that you know who you should contact first if the individual's condition deteriorates. Relatives should also be asked whether they would like to be called out during the night and their wishes should all be documented clearly and accurately within the individual's notes. It is vital to know who to notify in the event of deterioration of a person's general condition, or that individual's death and when it is acceptable to make contact, that is, time of the day or night. Telephoning the wrong person at an inappropriate time (e.g. a frail, elderly wife/husband at 3am) may cause distress. Loved ones who wished to be notified of a person's death, or wanted to be present as the individual passes away, regardless of the time of day or night, might be very upset if they are not notified.

Do not assume that relatives will notify each other. Always check that the family member contacted will take responsibility for informing other family members. If relatives are present at the time of death, always ask if they wish to use the phone or if there is anyone they would like you to contact. This is particularly important if a relative/friend is there alone. It is essential that you remain calm and show compassion and empathy.

Family and friends may want to spend time with the individual at the time of death and afterwards. They should be fully supported to do this if they wish. Make a key staff member available and be prepared for different responses to death.

Offer refreshments and provide a quiet space. Any conversations or meetings with relatives should be free from interruption. Ensure that they are given clear information and the person knows what to do next and where they need to go. Answer any questions and check the person has understood. It is vital to make sure that information is given at the appropriate moment. Give the person time to collect their thoughts, talk about their feelings and deal with their distress before you ask sensitive questions and give information. Listen and let them talk about their relatives and their feelings. Ask for the support of senior colleagues whenever you need this.

Never expect all people to react in the same way, some may not wish to sit with the person as they die or stay with the deceased. The important thing is that the person is not left to die alone, and that any relatives are comforted if they choose not to stay in the room as death approaches and afterwards.

Relatives should know where to collect the death certificate (if this is not available to give to them at the time) and where and how to register the death. Straightforward, written instructions may be helpful and will give information that a distressed relative may have forgotten. Your manager will advise relatives and you can help by passing on any concerns or questions loved ones may have.

The deceased's property should be packed tidily and a list made. Your organisation should have a policy on the return of property including flowers, food, confectionery and drinks. If these are not returned and not requested, keep them in case they are required in the following few days. The use of black bin bags is not allowed. Rinse through any soiled clothing and put in a sealed bag; mention this to relatives as they may not wish to have such items returned to them – however, do not assume this.

Check that people are not leaving alone or driving if they are distressed. Wherever possible, it should be arranged for someone to accompany them, pick them up or meet them at home. However, if a person insists they wish to be alone respect this. Report to your manager and keep them informed at all times; they will be able to advise and assist relatives. Your manager may phone the person later to see if they arrived safely and need anything or anyone.

Evidence activity

Supporting relatives, friends and other carers

Draw up a checklist you can use to provide support to relatives, friends and other carers.

LO3 Be able to contribute to preparing deceased individuals prior to transfer

3.1 Follow agreed ways of working to ensure that the deceased person is correctly identified

In NHS hospitals and private nursing homes the personal care after death is the responsibility of a registered nurse, although this and the packing of the property may be delegated to a suitably trained healthcare assistant. The registered nurse is responsible for correctly identifying the deceased person and communicating accurately with the mortuary or funeral director (in line with local policy). In care homes without a registered nurse, the home manager is responsible for ensuring that professional carers are trained appropriately and that they have the relevant competence for the role.

Time to reflect

3.1 Transferring a person after death

Where would a person be transferred to after death and why?

Pack personal property, showing consideration for the feelings of those receiving it and in line with local policy. Discuss the issue of soiled clothes sensitively with the family and ask whether they wish them to be disposed of or returned.

Provide the family with written information on the processes to be followed after death, including how to collect the Medical Certificate of Cause of Death (MCCD), where to register the death and the role of the funeral director and bereavement support agencies. Be aware of the information available for relatives in their local area and the nurse's role in ensuring that written information is given in a supportive way. Offer to guide people through its content and give them the opportunity to ask questions.

Evidence activity

3.1 The importance of identifying a person correctly

Explain why it is important that a person is identified correctly.

3.2 Carry out agreed role in preparing the deceased individual in a manner that respects their dignity, beliefs and culture

People react very differently after their loved one has died. Some may want to spend time with the person who has died, while others may not want to see them at all. There is no right or wrong way to feel or to act following the death.

The term used to describe the care given to an individual following their death is 'last offices'. It is the last thing that you will do for the individual. Your workplace will have policies and procedures on caring for the individual after death. The performance of last offices should take the following into account:

- dignity and privacy of the individual – screen the area, cover the body and only expose areas that need to be washed
- respect for the religious and cultural beliefs of the person/resident and their family
- appropriate care of bereaved relatives
- appropriate support for staff
- appropriate support for other people
- protection of staff, other people and relatives from infection and hazards
- care and safe custody of the property of the deceased
- compliance with policies, procedures and legal requirements.

Time to reflect

3.2 Policies and procedures that refer to preparing a person after their death

Which policies and procedures refer to preparing a person after their death?

It is essential that the individual can clearly be identified following death. It is vital that all documentation is accurate and, following your workplace policy, the body is clearly labelled. This could be achieved by attaching identity bands around the wrist and ankles. If you are responsible for performing last offices, you should also attach a notification of the death certificate to the sheet in which the individual is wrapped and clothing they are wearing.

Last offices refer to the final care acts of washing the body after the person's death and preparing it for removal. The procedures involved in last offices will depend on your care organisation's policy, although generally last offices will involve the following:

- Always find out, before touching the body, whether there are any religious or cultural rituals with regard to last offices. Do not proceed until you are sure.
- Last offices should not commence until death has been confirmed.

Two members of staff should undertake last offices:

- Wearing apron and gloves wash the body.
- Comb and style hair and ensure nails are clean and cut.
- Dress the person in a night garment, a shroud or any clothes they or the family have chosen.
- Take advice on any medical equipment, etc. It will depend on the circumstances of the person's death whether these need to be removed, replaced or left. Leaking wounds should be dressed and secured.
- Ensure the mouth is cleaned and any dentures are clean and replaced. Make sure the mouth and eyes are closed. The person may have made some requests with regard to jewellery, i.e. whether it is to be worn or given to relatives.
- Ensure all bed linen is replaced. If the person is to be viewed by relatives following last offices do not cover the face with a sheet. Make sure the relative can touch or hold the person's hand if they wish to.
- Remember to always preserve the person's dignity and privacy even after death.

Record all aspects of care after death in nursing and medical documentation and identify the professionals involved. Update and organise the medical and nursing records as quickly as possible so they are available to the bereavement team and other interested professionals, such as pathologists.

Research and investigate

(3.2) Offering dignity and privacy to a person

How can you offer dignity and privacy to a person?

Christianity

There are many different practices of Christianity, and each takes a different approach to their teachings and reflects different traditions of discussion and interpretation of the Bible.

A very sick person or a member of their family may ask a priest to visit as the individual is approaching death. The priest may perform one or more of the holy sacraments. By anointing the sick with oil in Christ's name, the priest asks him to alleviate suffering and heal the person, in this or the eternal life. The dying person may also want to take confession and Holy Communion. These rituals are important preparations for the individual's journey to the next life.

Care staff should be sensitive to the needs of the individual and their visitors. It is a good idea for the individual to be allocated a side room so that visitors can say prayers and sing hymns without disturbing others.

Judaism

If the individual is of Jewish faith, it is important that the individual's Rabbi is contacted. It is usual for relatives or friends to keep vigil by the body and recite prayers. It is important to respect their wishes and accommodate this as far as is possible.

It is essential that the body be laid flat, with hands open, arms parallel and close to the body, and the legs stretched out straight. There is no need to remove identification bracelets or wash the body, as the Jewish Burial Society will prepare it for burial. The body should then be wrapped in a sheet and removed to the appropriate place, according to your workplace policies and procedures.

A Jewish burial should take place as soon as possible after death and arrangements for the release of the body should be made without delay.

Hinduism

It is common for the family to stay near the bedside and be involved in the care of their relative as death approaches. They may also insist on the person's eldest son being present before, during and after death, even if he is a small child. It is important to the person that all close family members are present. It is also common for a Hindu priest to pray with the dying person and relatives to help the soul pass into another body. A blessed thread may be tied around the neck or wrist of the individual, and holy water is usually sprinkled over the person or used to wet their lips.

It is vital if death is imminent that the family are aware so that they can carry out rituals that are important to their faith. Any jewellery or religious object on the individual should not be removed from the body.

Some Hindus are very strict about who touches the body after death, and some families may feel distressed if a non-Hindu touches it. Close family members usually wash the body and their wishes to do this must be respected. The eyes are closed and legs straightened. The hair or beard must never be trimmed without first checking with the family.

The death of an individual of Hindu faith needs to be registered as soon as possible, and the body cremated within 24 hours. Many people may wish to pay their last respects to the individual, as this is a compulsory duty and should always be accommodated. The eldest son or another male relative traditionally prepares the body for burial and deals with the funeral arrangements.

Islam

Muslims believe in life after death and that when they die they will be judged by their actions. Good deeds will be repaid by everlasting life in heaven and bad deeds with everlasting life in hell.

When dying, privacy is important while the person declares their faith. Sometimes they are comforted by a recital from the Quran. It is important that you do not touch the body if you are a non-Muslim. Someone of the same sex within their family generally prepares the body. If you need to touch the body, you must use disposable gloves. The body must be released as soon as possible, as Muslims try to bury the body within 24 hours of death if possible. They believe that the soul departs at the moment of death.

Ritual washing is performed usually by family members or close friends, according to the sex of the deceased. The body is wrapped in a shroud of simple, white material. Afterwards prayers are said for the individual. Funerals are kept simple and respectful and it is forbidden to cremate the body of a Muslim.

Muslims are buried with their face turned to the right, facing Makkah ('Mecca' – The Holy City) and it is customary not to use a coffin. There is an official mourning period of three days (longer for a remaining spouse) and this may include a special meal to remember the individual.

Sikhism

People who follow the Sikh religion believe that the soul re-enters the cycle of birth and death after they have died, taking on different life forms depending on their actions in the former life. This religion has a symbolic dress code that is often referred to as the five Ks. This is because each item begins with the letter 'K':

- Kesh is uncut hair – Sikhs believe that hair should never be cut and should be left to grow as God intended. Many Sikhs keep their hair covered with a turban. Men should not cut their beard or moustache.
- Kangha – this is a small wooden comb used by Sikhs to keep their hair clean and tidy. Sikhs are encouraged to wash their hair daily and to comb it and wind it up into a topknot. The Kangha is then placed in the topknot to keep it in place.

- Kara – this is a bangle made out of steel or iron, which is always worn on the right wrist. The metal symbolises strength and the circle symbolises unity and eternity. It is a reminder of the Sikh's bond with the guru.
- Kirpan – this is a short sword or dagger. It is worn as a reminder of the courage of the first five Sikhs who were willing to die for their faith. It is a symbol of bravery and of faith in God. It is worn on a belt which goes across the shoulder under the clothes. Taking the Kirpan out of its sheath is considered disrespectful by some Sikhs.
- Kachera – these are short trousers that are worn under clothing and are worn by both men and women.

You should not disturb these symbolic items without permission, or before washing your hands. Non-Sikhs are permitted to care for the body of the deceased and healthcare staff may perform normal last offices, remembering not to interfere with the five Ks and, crucially, not to cut or trim hair from the face or head. Most relatives prefer to carry out these tasks themselves, but this should never be assumed.

It is normal that individuals have many visitors, this is seen as a mark of respect, and as many friends and relatives will visit the individual as possible. It may be helpful if the individual has a separate room in order to avoid disturbing others.

Friends and relatives are likely to visit and pray for a gravely ill individual. As there is no formal structure or hierarchy, someone such as an elder may approach staff to request administering last rites to the dying person. Others may wish to avoid touching a dead body, as to do so would require them to shave off their hair. Staff should be sensitive to the wishes of the person and their family, as there are no firm rules on who should carry out specific duties.

Sikhs may be comforted by reciting passages from Guru Granth Sahib. If they are too ill, a relative or someone from the local temple may be asked to read, which will be done quietly and should not disturb others. Holy water from the Gurdwara may be given to sip or be sprinkled on or around the person.

After death the body may be viewed several times before the funeral, so care should be taken to ensure that the eyes and mouth are closed and the facial expression is peaceful. Almost without exception, Sikhs are cremated and this should take place as soon as possible. If a delay is likely, the family should be given a full explanation.

Buddhism

Because rebirth is a fundamental part of Buddhism, the preparation for death prevails over the rituals associated with death. There is no one Buddhist death ritual, type of funeral or after-life requirement.

Buddhists who are facing death may request that a monk or nun be present to chant or assist in the passing from this life. Some traditions have special needs as death approaches. To assist in the passage to the next rebirth, which is not the same as reincarnation, wholesome acts such as generosity, service, kindness or pleasant thoughts are recalled.

However, in some traditions, it is desirable for the body to remain at the place of death for up to seven days to allow rebirth to occur. This may be a problem, but again Buddhists are noted for their tolerance, calmness and moderation, rather than for making demands, and usually a solution can be found.

Buddhists often opt for cremation, as the body is considered a vehicle that is temporary.

Evidence activity

 Finding out about the choices and beliefs of a specific religion

You are unsure of the choices and beliefs of a specific religion. How can you find out what should be done?

 Use protective clothing to minimise the risk of infection during preparation of the deceased individual

When a person dies standard infection control precautions are given a high priority and should be followed at all times, ensuring the safety of all persons who may come in contact with the person. PPE is worn to protect staff from body fluids to reduce the risk of transmission of infection between residents and staff and from one patient to another. The level of PPE used will vary based on the procedures being carried out and not all items of PPE will always be required.

Using personal protective equipment

Surgical masks may be used in a single episode for up to five hours provided the integrity of the mask is not compromised; for example, the mask provides a physical barrier which becomes ineffective once wet. As masks may become a reservoir for infection, hand hygiene must be performed after their removal and disposal. Masks should always be the last item of PPE to be removed.

Surgical masks should:

- cover both the nose and mouth
- not be allowed to dangle around the neck
- not be touched during use
- be changed when they become moist
- be worn once and discarded as clinical waste.

Gloves should be removed immediately after use, disposed of as clinical waste and hand hygiene performed.

A plastic apron:

- should be used to prevent contamination of staff uniform or clothing
- should be removed immediately after care is given, and discarded into a clinical waste bag
- should not be reused.

You should consider the use of a gown instead of an apron if extensive soiling of clothing or contact with blood or body fluids is anticipated.

Eye protection should be considered when there is a risk of contamination of the eyes with blood, body fluids, secretions or excretions.

Time to reflect

 PPE

When have you used PPE? Explain what you did and why.

It is vital that dignity, respect and religious preferences are observed when preparing a body for transfer to a funeral director/chapel of rest following death.

The circumstances of a death may need to remain confidential. Workers may be aware that the deceased has been suffering from a communicable disease. Registered and professional healthcare staff will be aware of their professional codes of conduct to maintain confidentiality. All other staff must be aware of relevant guidance relating to confidentiality.

Evidence activity

 A procedure for the correct use of PPE in your setting

Record a procedure for the correct use of PPE in your setting.

Evidence activity

 Explain how and where you should record a person's property

How and where should you record a person's property?

3.4 Contribute to recording any property and valuables that are to remain with the deceased individual

It is vital to follow policies and procedures to ensure the individual's property is stored safely. Check whether the individual has made any requests about jewellery: for example, whether it is to be worn or given to relatives.

At the appropriate time and as soon as possible write up all the necessary records as the workplace policy/operational procedure requires.

LO4 Be able to contribute to transferring deceased individuals

4.1 Carry out agreed role in contacting appropriate organisations

Table 8.5 sets out which practitioners can legally verify and which practitioners can certify death.

Table 8.5 Verification and certification of death

Who can legally verify death?	Who can legally certify death?
A medical practitioner will usually verify the death of an individual, but in cases where death is expected, and there are do not resuscitate orders in place (which should be clearly documented within the medical and nursing notes), some senior nurses can verify the death of an individual. This is also extended to some nursing and residential care homes.	The law states that a doctor must certify death. Usually the registered medical practitioner who attended the individual during their last illness certifies the death. If the individual dies in the community, either at home or within residential care, the GP should issue a medical certificate. If the death took place in hospital, depending on the time of death, the relatives may have to return the following day to pick up the medical certificate. Most hospitals have a special office for dealing with the bereaved. Returning to complete legal formalities can be very distressing for the bereaved, and relatives may need support. However, in the case of a hospice or care home, relatives may wish to return to speak with staff they have become close to and should, where appropriate, be invited to do so.

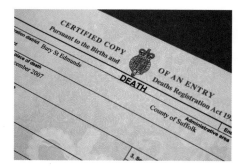

Figure 8.3 Paperwork

Prevention of hazards from cardiac pacemakers, and internal defibrillators

If an individual has a pacemaker, the mortuary staff and, if appropriate, the bereavement office should be informed. Always check with the person in charge. The presence of a cardiac pacemaker should be documented on the death notice. Written consent is required from relatives before a pacemaker is removed. The crematorium will require a certificate stating that the pacemaker has been removed before a cremation can take place.

If an individual has an internal defibrillator, the same procedure must be followed. The hazard here, however, is somewhat different. There is a risk of being shocked while handling the body. The defibrillator can be switched off externally by a special computer.

Human Tissue Act 2004

Although organ donation is normally associated with Intensive Care, it is not something to be ruled out in other areas. An individual may express that they would like to help someone else following their death, and it may be helpful if you know what to do in these circumstances.

The Human Tissue Act (HTA) 2004 replaced the Human Tissue Act 1961, the Anatomy Act 1984 and the Human Organ Transplants Act 1989 as they relate to England and Wales, and the corresponding Orders in Northern Ireland.

The Human Tissue Act 2004 covers England, Wales and Northern Ireland. It established the HTA to regulate activities concerning the removal, storage, use and disposal of human tissue. Consent is the fundamental principle of the legislation and underpins the lawful removal, storage and use of body parts, organs and tissue. Different consent requirements apply when dealing with tissue from the deceased and the living. The Human Tissue Act 2004 lists the purposes for which consent is required (these are called Scheduled Purposes).

There is separate legislation in Scotland – the Human Tissue (Scotland) Act 2006. While provisions of the Human Tissue (Scotland) Act 2006 are based on authorisation rather than consent, these are essentially both expressions of the same principle.

The key points of the Human Tissue Act 2004 are set out below. The Human Tissue Act 2004:

- regulates the removal, storage and use of human tissue – this is defined as material that has come from a human body and consists of, or includes, human cells

- creates a new offence of DNA 'theft' – it is unlawful to have human tissue with the intention of its DNA being analysed, without the consent of the person from whom the tissue came

- makes it lawful to take minimum steps to preserve the organs of a deceased person for use in transplantation while steps are taken to determine the wishes of the deceased, or, in the absence of their known wishes, obtaining consent from someone in a qualifying relationship.

Offences under the Human Tissue Act 2004 are:

- removing, storing or using human tissue for Scheduled Purposes without appropriate consent

- storing or using human tissue donated for a Scheduled Purpose for another purpose

- trafficking in human tissue for transplantation purposes

- carrying out licensable activities without holding a licence from the HTA (with lower penalties for related lesser offences such as failing to produce records or obstructing the HTA in carrying out its power or responsibilities)

- having human tissue, including hair, nails, and gametes (i.e. cells connected with sexual reproduction), with the intention of its DNA being analysed without the consent of the person from whom the tissue came or of those close to them if they have died. (Medical diagnosis and treatment, criminal investigations, etc., are excluded.)

The first four offences only apply in England, Wales and Northern Ireland, although the Human Tissue (Scotland) Act 2006 has similar offences and penalties. The offence of DNA theft applies UK-wide.

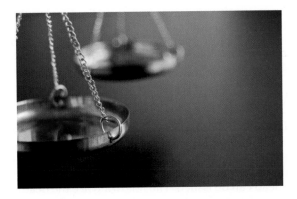

Figure 8.4 The Human Tissue Act 2004

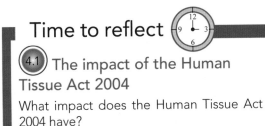

Time to reflect

4.1 The impact of the Human Tissue Act 2004

What impact does the Human Tissue Act 2004 have?

Registering the death

When someone dies, the doctor who was treating the deceased will issue a medical certificate of cause of death to the relatives. The person who will be registering the death must take this certificate to the registrar's office. Occasionally, if the death was sudden or the doctor treating the deceased is unavailable, it may not be possible for a medical certificate of cause of death to be issued. If this happens, the death will have to be reported to the coroner, which may lead to a delay in registering the death.

The registration of the death is the formal record of death and is carried out by the registrar of births, deaths and marriages. The address of the nearest registry office can be found in the telephone directory.

Relatives are required to register the death within five days. If the death has been reported to the coroner it is not possible to register the death until the coroner's investigations are finished.

The information required by the registrar in order that the death can be registered, includes:

- the date and place of death
- the name and address of the deceased
- maiden surname, if the deceased was a woman who had married
- the date and place of birth of the deceased
- the occupation or last known occupation of the deceased
- the deceased's marital status
- name and occupation of husband, where the deceased was a married woman or widow
- the date of birth of any surviving spouse
- usual address
- whether the deceased was in receipt of a pension or allowance from public funds.

When relatives are registering a death they must ensure that they take the following items:

- Medical certificate of cause of death
- The deceased's medical card, if available
- Birth certificate
- Marriage certificate, if applicable
- Pension book, if applicable
- Life insurance policies, if applicable.

It is most important that the information recorded in the death register is correct. If any mistake is made, for example, in the spelling of a name or surname, or in the description of the occupation, it will be difficult for the relative or other person who registered the death to have it put right. The person registering the death should check the information in the register very carefully before the entry is signed.

If English is not the first language of the relative or other person registering the death and assistance is needed, it would be helpful for someone else to accompany the person to the registrar's office and act as interpreter. However, the relative or other person must register the death personally, as a helper cannot register instead of them.

Every death in England or Wales must be registered in the district in which it takes place, within five days of the date of death. Information for the registration is given to the registrar by the person registering the death. The information, which is usually recorded on computer, is also recorded in the death register and the person registering the death signs the record.

If it is inconvenient for the person registering the death to go to the district where it took place, the information for the registration may be given to a registrar in another district. The registrar will record the registration particulars on a form of declaration and send it to the registrar for the district where the death occurred. The registrar who receives the declaration will enter the information in the death register. Certificates of the death, which may be ordered and paid for at the time of making the declaration, as well as the document allowing the funeral to proceed, will be posted to the person registering the death by the registrar for the district where it took place. If the declaration procedure is used, it may take a day or two longer for the document allowing the funeral to proceed to be issued. Relatives should discuss the arrangements with their funeral director and the registrar so as to avoid any delay to the funeral.

The registration of a death in Wales may be made bilingually in English and Welsh if the person who registers the death gives the information in Welsh and the registrar is able to understand and write Welsh. If the registrar cannot understand and write Welsh, the registration may be carried out in a different district where there are Welsh-speaking registrars, using the declaration procedure as described above. A death that takes place in England may be registered in English only.

The main Act and regulations governing the registration of births and death are:

- Births and Deaths Registration Act 1953 (as amended)
- The Registration of Births and Deaths Regulations 1987 (as amended)
- The Registration of Births and Deaths (Welsh Language) Regulations 1987 (as amended).

The people who can register a death fall into two slightly different categories, depending on whether the death occurred in a house or hospital, etc, or elsewhere. See Table 8.6.

The majority of deaths are registered by a relative of the deceased. The registrar would normally allow one of the other listed persons to register the death only if there were no relatives available.

Which deaths need to be reported to the coroner?

A small number of deaths have to be reported to the coroner before they can be registered and before the document allowing the funeral to go ahead can be issued. The following are the deaths that, if not already reported to the coroner by someone else, will be reported by the registrar:

- where there is no doctor who can issue a medical certificate of cause of death, or
- where the deceased was not seen by the doctor issuing the medical certificate after death, nor within 14 days before death, or
- where the cause of death is unknown, or
- where the cause of death is believed to be unnatural or suspicious, or
- where the death occurred during an operation or before recovery from an anaesthetic, or
- where the death is due to industrial disease or industrial poisoning.

Once a death has been reported to the coroner, the registrar cannot go ahead with the registration until the coroner has decided whether any further investigation into the death is necessary. In the vast majority of cases no further investigation is necessary and the registration can be completed straightaway.

Table 8.6 **People who can register a death**

Deaths in a house or hospital, etc.	Deaths elsewhere
• a relative of the deceased	• a relative of the deceased
• someone present at the death	• someone present at the death
• the occupier of the house or hospital if he or she knew of the death	• someone who found the body
• another person living at the house if he or she knew of the death	• a person in charge of the body
• the person making the arrangements with the funeral directors	• the person making the arrangements with the funeral directors

Which certificates will be issued?

The certificates issued by the registrar are given in Table 8.7

Table 8.7 Certificates issued by the registrar

The registrar will issue the following certificates:	
Death certificate	After a death has been registered, one or more certificates may be bought at the time of registration or at any time afterwards. You can obtain further information about obtaining certificates.
Certificate for burial or cremation	The registrar will issue a certificate for the burial or cremation of the body, which is normally passed to the funeral director by the relative who is making the arrangements. A funeral cannot proceed until this certificate is given to the burial authority or the crematorium. If there is a delay to the registration of the death, it is possible for a certificate for the burial of the deceased's body to be issued before registration, provided the death does not need to be reported to the coroner. A certificate for cremation cannot be issued before the registration of the death. If a death has been reported to the coroner, they may issue a certificate for burial or cremation where possible.
Certificate for applicable Social Security benefits	A certificate for sending to the Department of Social Security will also be issued by the registrar to the person registering the death or other applicant. The form serves a dual purpose; details of the death are given on one side and the other side is the application for applicable claim forms.

If a body is to be taken out of England and Wales, notice must be given to the coroner for the area where the body is lying. There is no restriction on the removal of bodies within England and Wales, but notice is necessary where the removal is to Scotland, Northern Ireland, the Isle of Man and the Channel Islands, as well as abroad.

A Form of Notice (form 104) may be obtained from a registrar or a coroner. Any certificate for burial or cremation already issued by the registrar or the coroner must be given to the coroner with the notice.

The coroner will acknowledge receipt of the notice and say when the removal of the body may take place. This will normally be after four clear days from when the coroner received the notice. If it is urgent, the person giving notice to the coroner should speak to them personally, since it may be possible to allow the removal sooner than the four days.

It is a criminal offence not to register a death, and you cannot delegate the responsibility for registering a death to someone else.

Once the death has been registered, the registrar then supplies a certificate for burial or cremation. This is known as a green form.

The death certificate is a copy of the entry made by the registrar in the deaths register. This certificate is needed to deal with any money or property left by the person who died, including dealing with a will.

Research and investigate

 Find out what information is included in a death certificate

What information is included in a death certificate?

Post mortem examinations – coroners' cases

A coroner is usually a doctor or a lawyer employed by a local authority to investigate certain deaths. Coroners are obliged to investigate sudden deaths, any death where the cause is uncertain and any death from unnatural causes. The coroner's job is to investigate the cause and circumstances of death and to ascertain the identity of the person who died. If the death has been referred to the coroner then relatives will not be issued with a medical certificate from the registrar or GP, but the coroner will issue his own disposal certificate.

When a death is reported to the coroner four courses of action are available:

- The coroner will advise that an ordinary medical certificate of death be issued by the doctor.
- The coroner will review the case but decide that no post mortem is necessary.
- The coroner will order a post mortem examination. The pathologist will then produce a written report stating the cause of death to the coroner.
- If the death is found to be of unnatural causes after a post mortem examination, an inquest will be arranged.

An inquest is a legal inquiry into the death of an individual. It is held in public, and relatives and friends can go along if they wish. Only a coroner can order an inquest. Relatives have no right to insist on one. Where an inquest takes place, the coroner has the discretion to refuse to allow the individual to be cremated. In simple terms, the purpose of an inquest is to find out:

- who the dead person is
- when the person came by their death
- where the person came by their death
- how the person came by their death.

Once the inquest is over the death can be registered and the funeral can take place.

Medical post mortem examinations

Medical post mortems can help doctors to understand more about why an individual may have died. If medical staff wish to carry out a post mortem they must ask permission from the next of kin. It is important that relatives are aware that they have every right to refuse a post mortem. This should be explained to them and they should never be put under any pressure to give their consent if they do not wish a post mortem to take place. The request for permission may cause distress to relatives and must be handled with great sensitivity. The doctor will make the request and then may leave the relatives to think about their decision. In these circumstances, the relatives may turn to you for support and reassurance.

However, if a coroner decides a post mortem is required, the relatives can do little. An application can be made to the Divisional Court, but these are rarely upheld. The coroner may request a post mortem for the following reasons:

- The doctor was not in attendance during the person's last illness.
- The doctor had not seen the dead person during the 14 days immediately prior to the death.
- The death may have been caused by an industrial disease.
- The deceased had served in the armed forces.
- The death was sudden or unexpected.
- The death was in suspicious circumstances.
- The death may have been caused by an accident.
- The death occurred in police custody or in prison.
- The death may have been related to an operation or to an anaesthetic.
- The death could have been due to neglect, self-neglect/poisoning, substance misuse.

Evidence activity

4.1 Explain the process that a post mortem follows

Research into the process that a post mortem follows and write an explanation of it.

 4.2 Carry out agreed role in transferring the deceased individual in line with agreed ways of working and any wishes expressed by the individual

The steps to be taken immediately after a death

Immediately following a death you will need to undertake the following steps:

- Notify the person in charge, who in turn should contact the person's GP or doctor to certify the death.
- Record the date and time of death and the people present.

- Contact the next of kin (if not present).
- Perform last offices according to personal and religious beliefs and any special requirements.
- Collect and record personal belongings ready to give to relatives.
- Support relatives in any way they need.

If you are unsure about what you should do following the death of an individual in your care, discuss your concerns with your manager.

When death occurs inform the medical practitioner primarily responsible for that person's care. Verification needs to be completed by a doctor or appropriately qualified nurse before the body is transferred from the care setting. Nurses need to be aware of local guidance regarding the criteria for verifying death, which should be in line with national guidance.

The privacy and dignity of the deceased on transfer from the place of death is paramount. Each organisation involved is responsible for ensuring that the procedures adopted to transfer bodies respect the values of personal dignity and that these are incorporated in the design of the concealment trolley and the way the body is covered. Place the body in an appropriate container to avoid causing distress to others. In community settings a funeral director will usually undertake transfer, although case law has determined that the deceased's executor (generally a family member) may also do this.

Follow standard infection control precautions during transfer and remove gloves when moving the body, as there is no risk of infection once the body is placed on the trolley. Try to retain a sense of the person's dignity in transit, avoiding busy public spaces if possible.

If the family are using a viewing room alongside a mortuary it is good practice for registered nurses to help them find it, ensure mortuary staff know to expect them and, if necessary, arrange for the family to be accompanied.

Evidence activity

(4.2) Iana

Iana has just died and you are in a rush to carry out last offices. Iana did have specific requirements and preferences in relation to her death. How can you find out what they are and why is it important to do so?

(4.3) Record details of the care and transfer of the deceased person in line with agreed ways of working

Record all aspects of care after death in nursing and medical documentation and identify the professionals involved. Update and organise the medical and nursing records as quickly as possible so they are available to the bereavement team and other interested professionals, such as pathologists.

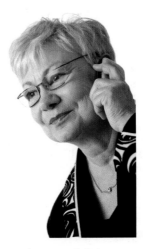

Figure 8.5 Roles and responsibilities

The person who provides the care after death takes part in a significant process, which has sometimes been surrounded in ritual. Although based on comparatively straightforward procedures, it requires sensitive and skilled communication, addressing the needs of family members/carers and respecting the integrity of the person who has died. It is a very difficult time for those who have been bereaved and can be emotionally challenging for nurses.

Care after death is a key responsibility for registered nurses in hospitals. In other settings (such as care and nursing homes, hospices and people's own homes) those responsible can also include carers, social care staff, GPs and funeral directors.

Professionals involved in this pathway include doctors, mortuary staff, hospital porters, ambulance staff, bereavement officers, police, social care staff, funeral directors, pathologists, coroners and faith leaders. Coordinated working between these individuals and organisations is vital if the process is to run smoothly.

Care after death includes:

- honouring the spiritual and cultural wishes of the deceased person and their family/carers while ensuring legal obligations are met
- preparing the body for transfer to the mortuary or the funeral director's premises
- offering the family and carers present the opportunity to participate in the process and supporting them to do so
- ensuring the privacy and dignity of the deceased person is maintained
- ensuring that the health and safety of everyone who comes into contact with the body is protected
- honouring people's wishes for organ and tissue donation
- returning the deceased person's possessions to their relatives.

■ Research and investigate

4.3 **Which practitioners are involved in this stage after death?**

Which practitioners are involved in this stage after death?

The nature of the death and the context in which it has occurred affects how care is provided, as well as the level of support needed by those who have been bereaved.

For example, some deaths are expected or peaceful, while others may be sudden or traumatic. As a result, families and carers are likely to have a range of responses and needs and each may also have differing views about how the person should be cared for after death. They may be very protective of the deceased person, feeling that their loved one has 'suffered enough'. Appropriate and sensitive nursing care at this time is therefore vital.

Record verification of death, the date and time this occurred in the notes and/or care pathway documentation, along with the name and contact details of the responsible practitioner. Be aware of local policy regarding nurses who are able to verify death.

The professional verifying the death is responsible for confirming the identity of the deceased person (where known) using the terminology of 'identified to me as'. This requires name, date of birth, address and NHS number (if known). It is good

practice for the person verifying the death to attach name bands with this information to the wrist or ankle of the deceased person. The following details are required when reporting a death to the coroner: the professional's telephone/bleep number; the deceased person's name, address, date of birth and GP details; family members' names, contact details and relationship to the deceased person; date and time of death; details of the person who pronounced life extinct and details of what happened leading up to the death.

The practitioner who verified the death ascertains whether the person had a known or suspected infection and whether this is notifiable. In such cases, they should then follow their local infection control policy regarding reporting responsibilities. It is vital that processes are in place to protect confidentiality, which continues after death. However, this does not prevent the use of sensible rules to safeguard the health and safety of all those who may care for the deceased. There needs to be clear communication regarding infection risk and the presence of implantable devices to mortuary staff and funeral directors. If the case is being referred to the coroner, seek advice before interfering with anything that might be relevant to establishing the cause of death. If the relatives or carers are not present at the time of death they need to be informed by a professional with appropriate communication skills and offered support, including access to a spiritual leader or other appropriate person.

When the death is unexpected, the health or social care professionals involved in caring for the person when they died need to inform the family face to face (whenever possible). They need the necessary communication skills to do this and to ensure there is appropriate support – such as an interpreter service – available where there may be communication barriers. They need to be aware of the physical environment and the needs of any children present. Adults may require guidance on how best to convey the news to children who are not present. If the deceased person was living in a care home but died in hospital, inform the home too, because staff may know about the person's wishes around death.

The police can be of assistance in locating relatives and breaking significant news.

The deceased was once a living person and therefore needs to be cared for with dignity. It is helpful if the surrounding environment conveys this respect. This includes the attitudes and behaviour of staff, particularly as bereaved people can experience high levels of anxiety and/or depression. Evidence suggests that the wider end of life care environment – for example, the journey to the mortuary and how the deceased's possessions are handled – not only has an immediate impact on relatives but also impacts on their subsequent bereavement.

The personal care after death needs to be carried out within two to four hours of the person dying, to preserve their appearance, condition and dignity. It is important to note that the body's core temperature will take time to lower and therefore refrigeration within four hours of the death is optimum. Tasks such as laying the deceased flat (while supporting the head with a pillow) and preparing them and the room for viewing need to be completed as soon as possible within this time. When families cannot view the body on a hospital ward, make arrangements for viewing at another appropriate location, such as a viewing room attached to a mortuary. In community settings there may be more flexibility for viewing arrangements.

Residents in communal settings, such as care homes and prisons, have often built up significant relationships with other residents and members of staff. Consider how to address their needs within the boundaries of patient confidentiality. If the person has died in an environment where other people may be distressed by the death then sensitively inform them that the person has died, being careful not to provide information about the cause and reason for death. Consider signposting to bereavement support in these settings.

Pack personal property showing consideration for the feelings of those receiving it and in line with local policy. Discuss the issue of soiled clothes sensitively with the family and ask whether they wish them to be disposed of or returned.

Provide the family with written information on the processes to be followed after death, including how to collect the MCCD, where to register the death and the role of the funeral director and bereavement support agencies. Be aware of the information available for relatives in their local area and the nurse's role in ensuring that written information is given in a supportive way. Offer to guide people through its content and give them the opportunity to ask questions.

Unless the death is suspicious and needs referring to the coroner and police, let the family sit with their relative if they wish in the period immediately after death. Offer age-appropriate support; for example, parents may wish a bereaved child to take a favourite toy to the hospital viewing room/funeral directors. Even after a traumatic death, relatives need the opportunity to view the deceased person and decide which family member, if any, should identify the body. Prepare them for what they might see and explain any legal reasons why the body cannot be touched. It should be noted that many mortuary staff have advanced skills in reconstruction and bodies may be more acceptable for viewing after post-mortem examination, though relatives need to know that the capacity for such reconstruction will differ greatly from case to case. Discussion with local mortuary staff on this issue can be valuable. Notify all other relevant professionals involved in the person's care that the person has died.

Evidence activity

 4.3 Important procedures that must be followed when completing records

Which important procedures must be followed when completing records?

LO5 Be able to manage own feelings in relation to the death of individuals

5.1 Identify ways to manage own feelings in relation to an individual's death

Grief may manifest itself in a number of ways

Grief serves the purpose of saying goodbye and letting go of the deceased, and until these are achieved, the individual who is grieving will be unable to move on in their lives.

Healthcare staff tend to build relationships with those for whom they care. When an individual they care for dies it is only natural that they will experience feelings of loss and grief. It is important for healthcare staff to acknowledge these feelings and not ignore them; otherwise they are in danger of becoming 'burnt out' and will therefore be unable to support others who are grieving.

Many organisations will have support systems in place for staff to express their feelings and work through their grief. Formal support systems include staff support groups or one-to-one supervision with a senior member of staff. Counselling services should also be available for staff if required. Support may also come informally from colleagues during a chat over coffee. It is important for any healthcare staff that talk about their feelings with family and friends to maintain confidentiality.

Some healthcare staff may prefer to express their feelings of grief by attending the funeral, or writing a letter of condolences to the family of the deceased.

Research and investigate

5.1 Find out how colleagues address their feelings following the death of a person they provide care for

Ask colleagues how they address their feelings following the death of a person they provide care for.

There will be a number of factors that will influence how long and how deeply felt grief is:

- whether there is a close relationship with the person who has died
- the individual's experience of loss during their lives
- support the grieving person has – their social networks
- religious or spiritual beliefs
- the age and gender of the person who is grieving
- if there has been any trauma or disease causing disfigurement to the body
- whether the loss is sudden or expected
- the quality of the relationship immediately prior to death.

A person may feel the need to hide their feelings because they find emotions difficult to express, have been taught that showing emotion is not appropriate or they are being 'strong' for others who are grieving (e.g. their children or elderly parent).

Stress

Stress is the way that you feel when pressure is placed on you. A little bit of pressure can be quite productive, give you motivation, and help you to perform better at something. However, too much pressure, or prolonged pressure, can lead to stress, which is unhealthy for both the mind and body. Stress can affect people, emotionally, behaviourally, and physically.

Emotionally, a person suffering from stress may experience:

- feeling overwhelmed
- irritability
- feeling depressed
- intolerance of others
- aggressiveness and/or anger

- suspiciousness
- fussiness
- restlessness
- anxiety
- despondency
- loss of concentration and/or memory
- feelings of panic
- nightmares or disturbed dreams
- a feeling of loneliness
- frequent crying
- lack of interest in sex.

Behavioural changes as a result of stress include:

- eating more or less
- sleeping too much or too little
- isolating oneself from others
- procrastinating or neglecting responsibilities
- developing nervous habits (e.g. nail biting, pacing the floor)
- increased smoking
- increased alcohol consumption
- increased casual sex
- obsessive dieting
- grinding of teeth
- an eye tic
- finger or foot tapping
- frowning
- excessive concern with time – arriving late, being early
- loss of interest in personal appearance
- loss of sense of humour
- lethargy
- accident prone.

Physical symptoms associated with stress include:

- chest pains
- constipation or diarrhoea
- cramps or muscle spasms
- dizziness
- fainting spells
- nail biting
- pins and needles
- feeling restless
- sexual difficulties such as erectile dysfunction or a loss of sexual desire
- breathlessness
- muscular aches
- difficulty sleeping
- headaches

- dry mouth and/or throat
- indigestion
- nausea
- sudden weight loss or weight gain
- ulcers
- high blood pressure
- palpitations
- excessive sweating
- rapid breathing/irregular breathing
- tightness in the chest
- frequent colds and/or flu.

Evidence activity

 5.1 **Review the availability and accessibility of support to enable you to manage your feelings following a death**

What support is available to you to enable you to manage your feelings following a death? Review their availability and accessibility.

5.2 Utilise support systems to deal with own feelings in relation to an individual's death

Emotions associated with loss and grief

Emotions associated with loss and grief include:

- numbness
- denial
- pining
- sadness and depression
- guilt
- anger
- anxiety.

Feeling emotionally numb is often the first reaction to loss; this can last a few hours, days or even longer. It is thought that this is a coping mechanism which can help individuals to get through the practical arrangements and family pressures that surround arranging a funeral. If this phase goes on for too long, it could lead to

problems in coping with life. It is important to realise that the shocked relative may not remember very much in the way of information around this time. However, they may remember vividly the way that the news was imparted.

Denial can help the bereaved person to cope with the loss for a short while, as they gradually absorb the fact that the death is real and final.

As the numbness and denial disappear, it may be replaced by a sense of yearning or pining for the dead person. The bereaved may feel a sense of the dead person's presence or may feel that the dead person is nearby and be desperate to find them. The bereaved person may experience sleep disturbances and bad dreams; they may even suffer from hallucinations (e.g. seeing the person who has died). They may need extra reassurance that they are not going insane during some of these experiences.

The bereaved person may suffer overwhelming sadness and may find they break down and cry frequently. They may find it difficult to cope with everyday activities, and may even attempt to withdraw themselves from social contact. It is important to recognise the signs and symptoms of clinical depression and to take action to obtain support for the individual affected.

Guilt is a common experience following bereavement. The individual may have certain regrets and may feel that they did not do enough for the dead person. This may be even more pronounced if the death was sudden, and the bereaved person did not get a chance to say goodbye. Those who have had to make a decision to withdraw life support, or stop or not commence treatment, may experience unbearable guilt.

Anger is a common feeling after the death of a loved one. It can be a confusing emotion, especially if it is directed at the dead person. Anger can take the form of blaming medical and nursing staff for not doing enough, or for failing to treat the illness. It is important to listen to individuals who address this anger towards staff. They may actually have a legitimate reason for complaint. A satisfactory outcome may help the bereaved in coming to terms with their grief. A danger may arise if the individual directs anger inwards, as this could lead to self-harm, self-neglect or suicide. Intervention may be necessary.

Anxiety and panic attacks may become apparent following bereavement. Prolonged and uncontrollable anxiety suggests that the bereaved individual may need professional help.

All emotions may be compounded if the deceased is perceived by those bereaved to have contributed in some way towards their own death (e.g. alcoholism, drug addiction, risk taking behaviour, suicide).

The phases of grief

The grieving process is very often described in stages, but it is important to realise that there are no definite stages where one phase begins and another one ends. This is because the stages are very much interlinked, and can change from day to day. It can be helpful, however, to be aware of the stages and to consider the fact that intense emotions and changes in mood are normal. See Table 8.8.

These various phases of the grieving process very often overlap and show themselves in different ways in different people. There is no definite time that this process should take. Each person will vary depending upon multiple factors. It is important to have knowledge of this in order for the care team to provide ongoing support. You may actually need to ask for support and guidance from other more experienced members of the healthcare team. It is essential that you recognise when you may need support. Observing and listening to the way that members of the care team support individuals may be of help to you.

Care staff should never be made to feel that they are being 'unprofessional' by showing signs of grief. If they hide their grief they are in danger of becoming 'burnt out', where the stress of dealing with the stressful aspects of palliative care are unsupported, and the person suffers stress, anxiety and loss of motivation which affects their personal and professional life.

There should be provision within your care organisation for staff to discuss and work through their grief. Referral to professional agencies should be available if a staff member is giving cause for concern.

Grief, which is an emotional response to loss, is an intensely personal reaction; but common elements are experienced in varying degrees by all bereaved individuals and are all normal components of the grieving process.

The time-scale of the grieving process varies considerably, and may be helped or hindered significantly by the amount of support available for the bereaved to help them explore their loss and continue with their lives.

Mourning is the outward expression of grief and is the process by which people adapt to loss. Cultural customs and rituals also influence the process.

Table 8.8 **Phases of grief**

Phase of grief	Effects on the individual
Initial	Within this stage, an individual may experience: **Psychological symptoms:** shock, sorrow, anxiety, distress, indecision, loneliness, insecurity, **Physiological/physical symptoms:** loss of appetite, nausea, feeling faint, increased heart rate, increased blood pressure, generally feeling unwell, fatigue, insomnia. **Cognitive changes:** poor concentration, memory impairment and loss of reality (daydreaming). A person may feel they hear the deceased person's voice or even see them. **Behavioural changes:** restlessness, agitation, crying, withdrawing from others and loss of interest in what is going on around them, their family, work, hobbies or friends. **Spiritual/religious:** a person may find comfort in their spiritual and religious beliefs and be able to make sense of their loss. Alternatively, the person may question their faith and belief system and feel confused and let down.
Middle	Within this phase of the process of grieving, the fierce pain of bereavement begins to fade. There is a decline of the initial emotions and physical symptoms. There is a readjustment to life without the loved one. However, the sense of having lost part of oneself never really goes away entirely. There is some attempt to return to the normality of life.
Resolution	The person going through bereavement remembers their loved one with fondness and pleasure and can now recall the good moments. This is the letting go of the person who has died and the start of a new sort of life.

Time to reflect

5.2 Other people's cultural customs

Which cultural customs do others adopt?

Unresolved grief

Although everyone grieves differently there will be certain parts of the grieving process that need to be worked through so the person can reach resolution. For some people they have great difficulty working through, and may remain 'stuck' somewhere in the grieving process.

Some people may not have had the opportunity to grieve properly. This could be for a number of reasons. They may have busy lives and lots of responsibilities. Other members of the family may have become reliant on that person to support them in their grief. This may lead to the grief reaction occurring sometime after the death. This is not necessarily a bad thing as it is a release for the person's feelings of grief and part of the healing process.

Sometimes people may start to grieve but become 'stuck' at some stage of the grieving process. This may be in the initial stage where the person remains shocked and in denial and the person may remain stuck in this stage for years.

Sometimes people may carry on with their life but be unable to think of very little else but their dead loved one. They may focus entirely on the dead person – affecting relationships with others as they, for example, refuse to clear the person's room, clothes or other possessions.

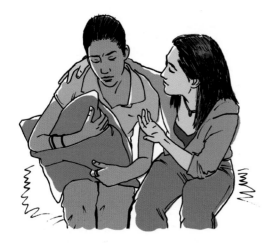

Figure 8.6 Unresolved grief

Unresolved grief can affect the person's life, relationship and mental health. Help can be given in the space of voluntary groups or care professionals such as counsellors.

Your feelings may seem unimportant as you support people who are dying and the bereaved on a daily basis. Acknowledging your own grief and stress may make you feel guilty, that it is not you who should feel this way. However, to avoid excess stress and burnout you must look after your own well-being:

- Take time out – discuss with your manager about having a designated quiet area where you and other staff can go for time to yourself. You need to be clear about when this is appropriate and the procedures for letting others know where you are and how long you will be gone. Taking time out at home may be helpful too.

- Discuss your feelings with others – colleagues, friends, family (ensuring confidentiality). Your manager may be able to arrange a support group within your care setting. You should be aware of counselling services, help lines, groups, etc.

- Grieve losses – acknowledge grief; cry if you want to (not in front of family) and talk over grief with colleagues. Mark the person's life.

- Try to find ways to relax while away from work – this will help you to reduce stress.

- Reward oneself – give yourself little treats and do what you enjoy. Never feel guilty because those you care for are going through suffering and you feel you shouldn't enjoy yourself. Improving everybody's quality of life is important and that includes you.

- Be aware of your own limitations – you are not expected to know everything and cope with every situation. Know your limits and ask for support.

Bereavement can be defined as 'a state of loss resulting from death'. Grief is 'the psychological and emotional reaction to bereavement' (C. Murray-Parkes, *Bereavement, Oxford Textbook on Palliative Medicine* (2001)). Mourning is the psychological process of adaptation to life without the person, including rituals and customs. It cannot be emphasised enough that grief is a natural response to human loss.

Evidence activity

 5.2 How does Cruse help bereaved people?

Cruse is a national charity set up to offer free, confidential help to bereaved people. How does it provide this help?

Assessment summary

Your reading of this chapter and completion of the activities will have prepared you to demonstrate your learning and understanding of end of life care. To achieve this unit, your assessor will require you to:

Learning outcomes	Assessment criteria
Learning outcome 1: Know the factors that affect how individuals are cared for after death by:	(1.1) outlining legal requirements and agreed ways of working that underpin the care of deceased individuals See Evidence activity 1.1, p.182
	(1.2) describing how beliefs and religious and cultural factors affect how deceased individuals are cared for See Evidence activity 1.2, p.185
	(1.3) identifying the physical changes that take place after death and how this may affect laying out and moving individuals See Evidence activity 1.3, p.186
	(1.4) identifying diseases and conditions that necessitate specialist treatment or precautions when caring for and transferring deceased individuals See Evidence activity 1.4, p.187
	(1.5) describing the precautions needed when undertaking the care and transfer of deceased individuals with specific high risk diseases and conditions See Evidence activity 1.5, p.188
Learning outcome 2: Be able to contribute to supporting those who are close to deceased individuals by:	(2.1) describing the likely immediate impact of an individual's death on others who are close to the deceased individual See Evidence activity 2.1, p.195
	(2.2) supporting others immediately following the death of the individual in ways that: • reduce their distress • respect the deceased individual See Evidence activity 2.2, p.196

Learning outcomes	Assessment criteria
Learning outcome **3**: Be able to contribute to preparing deceased individuals prior to transfer by:	(3.1) following agreed ways of working to ensure that the deceased person is correctly identified See Evidence activity 3.1, p.197
	(3.2) carrying out agreed role in preparing the deceased individual in a manner that respects their dignity, beliefs and culture See Evidence activity 3.2, p.200
	(3.3) using protective clothing to minimise the risk of infection during preparation of the deceased individual See Evidence activity 3.3, p.201
	(3.4) contributing to recording any property and valuables that are to remain with the deceased individual See Evidence activity 3.4, p.201
Learning outcome **4**: Be able to contribute to transferring deceased individuals by:	(4.1) carrying out agreed role in contacting appropriate organisations See Evidence activity 4.1, p.206
	(4.2) carrying out agreed role in transferring the deceased individual in line with agreed ways of working and any wishes expressed by the individual See Evidence activity 4.2, p.207
	(4.3) recording details of the care and transfer of the deceased person in line with agreed ways of working See Evidence activity 4.3, p.209
Learning outcome **5**: Be able to manage own feelings in relation to the death of individuals by:	(5.1) identifying ways to manage own feelings in relation to an individual's death See Evidence activity 5.1, p.211
	(5.2) utilising support systems to deal with own feelings in relation to an individual's death See Evidence activity 5.2, p.213

Good luck!

Web links

Alzheimer's Society	www.alzheimers.org.uk
Care Quality Commission (CQC)	www.cqc.org.uk
Cruse Bereavement Care	www.crusebereavementcare.org.uk
Department of Health	www.dh.gov.uk
Huntington's Disease Association	www.hda.org.uk
Macmillan Cancer Support	www.macmillan.org.uk
Marie Curie Cancer Care	www.mariecurie.org.uk
Multiple Sclerosis Society	www.mssociety.org.uk
National Council for Palliative Care	www.ncpc.org.uk
National End of Life Care Programme	www.endoflifecareforadults.nhs.uk
Parkinson's Disease Society	www.parkinsons.org.uk
The Motor Neurone Disease Association	www.mndassociation.org
Princess Royal Trust for Carers	www.carers.org

Glossary

Anticipatory grief refers to the emotions that dying people and their loved ones experience before death.

Anticipatory loss refers to the sense of loss experienced before a person dies.

Autonomy is the condition or quality of being autonomous or independent.

Bereavement is the state of being deprived of something or someone.

Braille is a form of written language for the visually impaired, in which characters are represented by patterns of raised dots that are felt with the fingertips.

Cheyne–Stokes breathing is an abnormal type of breathing seen especially in unconscious people, characterised by alternating periods of shallow and deep breathing.

Cognitive relates to the mental processes of perception, memory, judgment, and reasoning.

Collaborative means to work together in a joined up way.

Complementary therapies: the practice of medicine without the use of drugs; they may involve herbal medicines, self-awareness, biofeedback or acupuncture.

Coping strategies are the overall pattern of coping responses.

Cumulative grief can occur where unresolved grief from a number of bereavement experiences accumulates and causes a deep feeling of bereavement.

Dignity is concerned with respecting people for who they are and what they believe in.

Empathy means understanding and imaginatively entering into another person's feelings.

Genuine: to be genuine indicates honesty, integrity and a commitment to be truthful.

Gestures refer to the hand and head movements or signals which many people use to emphasise what they are saying.

Grief is the sadness a person feels, usually as a result of loss.

Holistic refers to the treatment of the whole person, taking into account mental and social factors, rather than just the physical.

Identity is the fact of being whom or what a person or thing is.

Ketoacidosis occurs when the body cannot use sugar (glucose) as a fuel source because there is no insulin or not enough insulin. Fat is used for fuel instead.

Mourn means to feel sorrow or express grief.

Non-judgemental relates to an attitude which is open and not incorporating a judgement one way or the other.

Palliative care is care that aims to enhance the quality of life of service users who are faced with a life limiting illness and their families. It focuses on increasing comfort through prevention and treatment of suffering.

Personal autonomy relates to being self-governing or independent.

Person centred: a person-centred approach will place the person at the centre of all discussions and decisions.

Proximity relates to the distance that is maintained between people throughout the process of communication.

Psychosocial means involving aspects of both social and psychological behaviour.

Reciprocity means responding to a positive action with another positive.

Taboo refers to a strong social prohibition (or ban) relating to any area of human activity or social custom that is sacred and forbidden based on moral judgment and religious beliefs.

Values are important and enduring beliefs or ideals shared by the members of a culture about what is good or desirable and what is not.

The World Health Organisation (WHO) is the directing and coordinating authority for health within the United Nations system. It is responsible for providing leadership on global health matters, shaping the health research agenda, setting norms and standards, articulating evidence-based policy options, providing technical support to countries and monitoring and assessing health trends.

Index

NORTHBROOK COLLEGE SUSSEX
LEARNING RESOURCE CENTRE
LIBRARY